Roselle Kurland, PhD
Robert Salmon, DSW
Editors

Group Work Practice in a Troubled Society: Problems and Opportunities

Pre-publication
REVIEWS,
COMMENTARIES,
EVALUATIONS . . .

"**T**his is a profoundly rich volume. In the choice of papers for *Group Work Practice in a Troubled Society*, editors Kurland and Salmon keep faith with the theme and purpose of the Fifteenth Annual Group Work Symposium which they chaired: to be reflective of the social realities in which group work is now practiced. This is an important addition to our field."

Sue Henry, DSW
Professor,
Graduate School of Social Work,
University of Denver

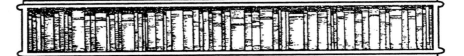

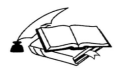

particular significance is the description of interdisciplinary work with a group of nurses working out their grief over sudden and/or unexpected death of patients. A model for stages of development in a women's group is also presented that suggests interesting gender differences.

This is an invaluable book, not only for social work education, but for the social work practitioner who is looking for innovative ways to deal with current social problems."

Celia B. Weisman, DSW
Professor Emerita,
Wurzweiler School of Social Work,
Yeshiva University

The Haworth Press, Inc.

Group Work Practice in a Troubled Society
Problems and Opportunities

PLANNING COMMITTEE
FOR THE
FIFTEENTH ANNUAL SYMPOSIUM
OF THE
ASSOCIATION FOR THE ADVANCEMENT OF SOCIAL WORK WITH GROUPS
New York City, October 21-24, 1993

Chairpersons
Roselle Kurland   Robert Salmon

Symposium Coordinator
Dominique Steinberg

The New York City Planning Group

Virginia Abrams	Martha Friedlaender	Laurel Meyer
Sylvia Aron	George Getzel	Irving Miller
Aaron Beckerman	Paul Gitelson	Manny Munoz
Martin Birnbaum	Alex Gitterman	Paula Nesoff
Dianne Bradford	Urania Glassman	Catherine Papell
Julie Stein Brockway	Mel Goldstein	Stephan Russo
Len Brown	Maxine Lynn	Florence S. Schwartz
Amy Chalfy	Eileen Lyons	Sally Ann Shields
Carol Cohen	Randy Magen	Celia Weissman
Dawn Cavrell Epstein	Andrew Malekoff	Bernard Wohl

Laura Mack - **Volunteer Coordinator**, Paula Nesoff - **Continuing Education Unit Coordinator**, Carol Cohen - **Hospitality Coordinator**, Josephine Hayes Dean - **Video Filming Coordinator**

Officers of the Board of Directors of AASWG - 1993

James A. Garland, *Chairperson, Boston University School of Social Work,* Boston, MA
Maxine Lynn, *Vice-Chairperson, Fordham University Graduate School of Social Service,* NYC
Paul H. Ephross, *Secretary, University of Maryland School of Social Work,* Baltimore, MD
Julianne Wayne, *Treasurer, University of Connecticut School of Social Work,* West Hartford, CT
John H. Ramey, *General Secretary, University of Akron,* Akron, OH

Group Work Practice in a Troubled Society
Problems and Opportunities

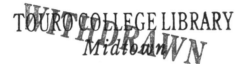
Roselle Kurland, PhD
Robert Salmon, DSW
Editors

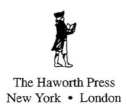

The Haworth Press
New York • London

MT

The Haworth Press, Inc., 10 Alice Street, Binghamton, NY 13904-1580

Library of Congress Cataloging-in-Publication Data

Group work practice in a troubled society : problems and opportunities / Roselle Kurland, Robert Salmon, editors.
    p. cm.
    Selected papers from the fifteenth annual Symposium of the Association for the Advancement of Social Work with Groups, held in New York City in October 1993.
    Includes bibliographical references and index.
    ISBN 1-56024-962-5 (alk. paper).
    1. Social group work. 2. Social service. 3. Social work education. I. Kurland, Roselle. II. Salmon, Robert, 1930-   . III. Association for the Advancement of Social Work with Groups. Symposium (15th : 1993 : New York)
HV45.G7314 1995
361.4–dc20
                                            95-14393
                                            CIP

6/25/08

CONTENTS

ABOUT THE EDITORS

Roselle Kurland, PhD, is a Professor at the Hunter College School of Social Work. She is Editor of the journal *Social Work with Groups* and serves as a consultant to a range of social agencies, working with staff to enhance their skills in group work practice and to develop creative programs. Dr. Kurland is a member of the Board of Directors of the Association for the Advancement of Social Work with Groups.

Robert Salmon, DSW, is a Professor at the Hunter College School of Social Work where he was Associate Dean and Acting Dean for a period of 16 years. He teaches Social Work with Groups and Administration and consults in both practice areas with a wide variety of social agencies. Dr. Salmon is active as a board member of social agencies and professional social work organizations, including a current term on the Board of the Association for the Advancement of Social Work with Groups.

Drs. Kurland and Salmon have been colleagues at Hunter College for 17 years. Their collaboration began in the early 1980s when they started to write and present together. They have coauthored a series of articles on the practice of teaching of group work.

Contributors

Cyrus S. Behroozi, PhD, Professor, Indiana University, School of Social Work.

Sondra Brandler, DSW, Adjunct Assistant Professor, Herbert H. Lehman College, Department of Sociology and Social Work.

Carol Pigler Christensen, PhD, Professor, The University of British Columbia, School of Social Work.

Elaine P. Congress, DSW, Assistant Professor, Fordham University Graduate School of Social Service.

Paul H. Ephross, PhD, Professor, School of Social Work, University of Maryland at Baltimore.

Hans S. Falck, PhD, Professor Emeritus, School of Social Work, Virginia Commonwealth University.

Maeda J. Galinsky, PhD, William R. Kenan Professor, School of Social Work, The University of North Carolina at Chapel Hill.

Judith Gillis, BN, RN, affiliated with the Public Health Nursing Office.

Kalev Helde, MSW, Social Worker, Family Services, Catholic Children's Aid Society of Metropolitan Toronto, Etobicoke Branch.

Patricia A. Joyce, ACSW, doctoral student at Hunter College School of Social Work, CUNY Graduate Center.

John KixMiller, MSW, Director of the After School Program, Center for Family Life, Brooklyn, NY.

Elizabeth A. Lewis, RN, CSW, Senior Clinical Supervisor, Ulster County Mental Health Department, Kingston Mental Health Center.

Fanny W. C. L. Liu, MSS, Senior Lecturer, Division of Humanities and Social Sciences, City Polytechnic of Hong Kong.

Maxine Lynn, CSW, Director of Field Education, Fordham University Graduate School of Social Service.

Paule McNicoll, PhD, Assistant Professor, The University of British Columbia, School of Social Work.

Ruth R. Middleman, EdD, Professor Emerita, Raymond A. Kent School of Social Work, University of Louisville.

Helene Filion Onserud, MSW, Social Worker, Center for Family Life, Brooklyn, NY.

Joan K. Parry, DSW, Professor Emerita, San Jose University School of Social Work.

Camille P. Roman, ACSW, in private practice, and Adjunct Assistant Professor, Hunter College School of Social Work.

Linda Yael Schiller, LICSW, Adjunct Assistant Professor, Boston University School of Social Work.

Janice H. Schopler, PhD, Associate Dean and Professor, School of Social Work, The University of North Carolina at Chapel Hill.

Neil Stokes, MSW, Social Worker, Sir Thomas Roddick Hospital, Newfoundland, Canada.

Jane Tanner, MSW, Medical Social Worker, San Jose Medical Center.

Harle Thomas, MEd, Coordinator for Support Groups at McGill University Sexual Assault Center.

Anna Travers, MSW, Opportunity for Advancement, Toronto, Ontario.

Joan C. Weiss, MSW, Executive Director, Justice Research and Statistics Association, Washington, DC.

Gale Goldberg Wood, EdD, Professor, Raymond A. Kent School of Social Work, University of Louisville.

Acknowledgment

We are pleased to acknowledge and express our gratitude to The Charles A. Frueauff Foundation for its support of Social Work with Groups.

Introduction

Roselle Kurland
Robert Salmon

With more than 800 persons attending and more than 50 sponsoring agencies and institutions, the Fifteenth Annual Symposium of the Association for the Advancement of Social Work with Groups (AASWG), held in New York City in October 1993, was the largest in the organization's history. The symposium was rejuvenating for the many veteran practitioners and educators who were present and eye-opening and exciting for the many newcomers who were attending their first group work symposium. It was four days of serious work and intense involvement in presentations, papers, and discussions, along with the fun and joy of meeting others who share common experiences, concerns, and interests.

In 1991, when the Board of Directors of AASWG first discussed its hopes for the Fifteenth Symposium, board members emphasized the importance of making the Symposium reflective of the social realities in which group work is now practiced and of including papers that would address the social issues and problems that social work and group work currently confront. In 1992, at its first meetings, the New York City Planning Group emphatically agreed. The theme, *Group Work Practice in a Troubled Society: Problems and Opportunities*, was selected and a call for papers was developed that emphasized the New York Group's intention to carry out this theme throughout the Fifteenth Symposium.

The New York City Planning Group also very much wanted the Fifteenth Symposium to provide a chance for active participant discussion and involvement. To accomplish this, a number of innovative symposium features were developed: Pre-Symposium Outstitutes, where small groups of participants looked at social work practice with HIV/AIDS clients, immigrants, or formerly homeless adults while also seeing New York City; Networking Sessions, where those interested in work with AIDS, issues of race/culture/ethnicity, and/or work with youth could meet for discussion of issues and ideas as well as support; an Author's Forum, where authors of papers dealing with a range of topics could make their manuscripts available to and interact informally with colleagues who shared similar interests. In addition, in a number of symposium sessions, the members of client groups demonstrated the kinds of activities in which they engage in their groups and/or discussed their group participation and its meaning for them; in other sessions, the audience was asked to learn through firsthand experience by participating in a range of activities.

Participants left the symposium with a sense of hope and renewal. And hope and renewal were very much needed. Ann Hartman recently wrote, "It is a difficult time to be a social work practitioner and . . . also it is a difficult time to be a social work educator" (1990). Social concerns continue to be low on a list of national priorities despite the fact that social problems are deepening and becoming more complex. Social programs have been decimated and resources are scarce. Middleman and Wood, in their chapter in this volume, cite a recent article (Strom and Gingerich, 1993) that presents the content that should be taught to social work students in light of "new market realities," realities forcing social agencies to become businesses concentrating on reimbursable services. Meanwhile, despite the fact that work with groups proliferates, social work students continue to be poorly educated in the area of group work practice as the curricula of schools of social work continue to include little about groups and group work practice.

Larry Shulman's announcement at the symposium that the Council on Social Work Education had agreed to work with AASWG to develop three teaching guides for the reintroduction of curricula on the teaching of group work practice in the classroom and in the field certainly contributed to the sense of hope and renewal. But perhaps most important, this symposium, as the others that preceded it, was a unifying event for those with a special interest in group work practice. The Fifteenth Symposium was a huge international gathering where practitioners and educators were inspired by the concerns and practice of colleagues and where the sense of professional isolation was diminished.

There were more than 150 presentations at the Fifteenth Symposium. From these rich examples of practice, 18 papers have been selected to represent the event. The authors include some longtime contributors to the conceptual and practice literature of social work, as well as some newcomers who have not published previously. They discuss innovations in practice, programs, and theory, and a wide variety of experiences with clients in many different settings. There is a range and strength and diversity in group work practice today, and these 18 contributions from practitioners and educators in the United States, Canada, and Hong Kong represent the vitality of practice and theory. We hope that the reader will find that this volume, too, is another sign of hope and renewal for the practice of group work today and continuing into the future.

REFERENCES

Hartman, Ann (1990). Education for Direct Practice. *Families in Society, 71*(1), 44-50.

Strom, Kimberly and Gingerich, Wallace J. (1993). Educating Students for the New Market Realities. *Journal of Social Work Education, 29*(1), 78-87. Cited in Ruth R. Middleman and Gale Goldberg Wood, Contextual Group Work: Apprehending the Elusive Obvious, in this volume.

Chapter 1

Contextual Group Work:
Apprehending the Elusive Obvious

Ruth R. Middleman
Gale Goldberg Wood

In this excursion into group work the term context has two meanings: on the one hand, context refers to the times–the political/so-
cial/economic situation in which the group is embedded; and on the
other hand, each group contains a multiplicity of contexts–the different specifics of living that each member brings. In both senses,
appreciating the impact of context in a postmodern world involves
new understandings of the influence of the situational surround and
of the institutional, ideological, and historical forces that press upon
the lives and perspectives of the group participants. Context is the
hub of this journey.

And what is the elusive obvious? Something that is obvious is
something that is easily understood. Something to which we are
oblivious is something outside of our conscious awareness. But
nothing is categorically obvious. And we are all too frequently
oblivious to this. This brings us to our second theme: the oxymoron,
elusive obvious. It is other people's meanings.

CONTEXT

In 1910 Teddy Roosevelt lamented the context for his work:
(One) has to take advantage of (one's) opportunities, but the
opportunities have to come. If there is not the war, you don't

get the great general. If there is not the great occasion, you don't get the great statesman. If Lincoln had lived in times of peace, no one would know his name now. (Brinkley, 1993)

The argument is that the times make the person. And what of our times? These are hostile times for social workers and for clients. These are times rife with violence, drugs, homelessness, and AIDS; one-third of our citizens are without health-care provision, and interest groups spar over what should be the national health plan; one child dies because of poverty every 53 minutes. These are times when an inner-city school where children *are* learning merits a news story; when a black man in Bangladesh has a better chance of living to age 65 than a black man in Harlem; and when one out of four girls is molested before she reaches her 18th birthday.

Ours is an era in which federal social programs are being eliminated or shuffled to the states or local communities, and no one wants to pay more taxes or imagine the human suffering of drastic cutbacks in funding. Clarke Chambers, noted social welfare historian and keeper of the social welfare archives, aptly titled his keynote address at the centennial celebration of the University of Chicago, "Uphill All the Way." In it he described the plight of workers in the human services and made the following observation:

> the Schlesingers claimed history is cyclical: reform, consolidation, reaction, growing unmet problems, and reform again . . . (but) there is no such cycle in the history of social welfare . . . American society has been prudent in the use of public funds, miserly in provision of assistance to vulnerable persons and groups, quick to blame victims for their plight, and deferential to property over personal rights . . . .(1992, 499)

Since human services are offered at the largess of society, social workers, along with those they serve, are vulnerable. As one student social worker at a family and children's agency wrote:

> There are therapy groups for both male and female adult survivors of sexual victimization. There are groups for child survivors and there are groups for perpetrators. There have never been groups for non-offending parents of sexually abused chil-

dren. The staff was very responsive to my offer to start a support group for them, however our director eliminated the word *support* in order that the participants could be charged a fee. So now the director and the staff expect it to be a therapy group, the members expect to be educated about child abuse, and I want it to be a support group emphasizing mutual aid among the group members. I have a lot to overcome to do the kind of group work I want to do.

We note with alarm the directives in a recent article in the *Journal of Social Work Education* regarding what should be taught to students in light of the "new market realities," realities forcing social agencies to become businesses. According to Strom and Gingerich (1993), these realities include: licensure and vendorship legislation; expansion of managed care and third-party payments; limits on which services are reimbursed and how they must be delivered; growth of for-profit institutions; results-oriented outcomes; emphasis on diagnosis, assessment, and treatment planning, and the pathology-oriented medical model; diagnostic labels; an assault on confidentiality; and involvement of managers from the funding source in determining the appropriate (reimbursable) services, which will likely exclude many children, the elderly, people living in poverty, minorities, and the more severely impaired.

Where is group work in all of this? It has largely succumbed to the pressures for containment and management of symptoms (Lewis, 1992). Garland reports on the proliferation of expedience-driven time-and-structure formats, truncated groups like the 35 minute hour typical of public school-based group work. Accordingly, workers hold increased power over group members, mutual aid gives way to programmed exercises, groups for sexual abuse and other traumas end before deeper aspects are considered, and detox groups decrease in length with every new budget cut (Garland, 1992).

In fact, it would be fair to say that *preposition* groups abound these days.

There are the *of* groups: victims of . . . ; perpetrators of . . . ; families of . . . ; adult children of . . .

There are the *from* groups: from Vietnam; from Russia; from Haiti; from Desert Storm; from Hurricane Andrew; from the flood of 1993.

There are the *with* groups: persons with AIDS; with cancer; with hypertension; with developmental disabilities.

There are the *in* groups: in prison; in mental hospitals; in recovery; in nursing homes; in trouble.

And there are the *for* groups: for codependent women; for managing stress; for dealing with burnout (as if the organization were not the appropriate target to be changed).

All of these preposition groups are constructed groups–groups of strangers collected because of one shared attribute they need to move beyond or learn to live with. These are the top-down groups with goals and processes determined for the participants by others. How different this context is from that of earlier times, when group workers dealt with natural groups devoted to socialization and development, and neighborhood groups for social action–bottom-up group work.

CONSTRUCTIVISM

Context is at the core of an approach to knowing called constructivism. According to constructivist thinking, understanding is a matter of interpretation by the experiencing person (von Glasersfeld, 1984). Some key aspects of constructivism are: all knowledge is constructed and the knower is an intimate part of the known (Goodman, 1984); objectivity is impossible in the human sphere (Gergen, 1991); language creates reality (Bruner, 1986); people are historically situated when they construct their views of reality (Weick, 1991); and people are the final arbiters of the meaning of their own experiences which they express in narratives or stories (Laird, 1989). There is no reality apart from one's construction of it in dialogue with others, and there are as many constructions of reality as there are experiencing person. Science itself is a construction (Guba and Lincoln, 1989)–one of many intellectual pursuits alongside of, but not above, literary criticism, jurisprudence, history, and so forth (Brown, 1992). No one is an expert on another's situation (Hoffman, 1990). And there is reason to wonder about the "extent to which we can really comprehend another's life" (Goldstein, 1990, 271).

Ideas about the world start with perception and form perspective. For many years we have studied perception and its implications for practice, distinguishing between perception and cognition (Middleman, 1985; Middleman and Goldberg Wood, 1990), between looking–a visual experience–and seeing–a cognitively embellished outcome of looking (Goldberg and Middleman, 1980; Middleman and Goldberg Wood, 1985; Middleman and Goldberg Wood, 1991). Constructivism is about how this connects to *knowing*.

Constructivist thinking has to do with how people look at things, seeing them differently. It is about ways in which they talk to each other about what they see, creating through such talk with others an agreement about how things are. Through such dialogues or conversations, people interpret their world. Individual interpretations merge with others to create an understanding of what is out there (Middleman and Goldberg Wood, 1994).

Thus, meaning is *socially* constructed (Berger and Luckman, 1967). It is local (Geertz, 1983), not universal; and of a particular era, not timeless. People's versions of reality also differ according to their location in the social structure. Their position creates their standpoint. Less powerful members of society experience a reality that reflects their oppression, a reality different from the experiences of more dominant people (Swigonski, 1993). To survive, the less powerful must have knowledge of and be sensitive to both the dominant group's view of society *and* their own, requiring *bicultural socialization*, "the ability to move freely between one's ethnic community and the larger culture" (Chau, 1990, 2). Bicultural socialization has been described in social work literature by DeAnda (1984) for minorities of color; by Lukes and Land (1990) for lesbians and gay men; by Bilides (1990) for teenagers in school; and by Van Den Bergh (1990) for employees in the workplace.

In our social work practice classes we have tried to help students confront their own differing constructions of meaning experientially by asking them to look at a poster with five bands of color–red, orange, white, green, and black–and to remove two colors that they believe least belong, and write their reason for the choice. They are surprised by the different rationales reported, even with such seemingly neutral stimuli as colors. The responses are especially impressive when there is at least one African-American student present. The Black African flag is there (red, black, green). Although the white students never see it, it is ordinarily *seen* by the African-American students, but not acknowledged until the instructor calls attention to it. In one instance, an African-American student firmly stated he would notice black and white first because these colors were uppermost in his thinking all the time, while the other students could think of other things. There followed a discussion of how it felt to be the only black person in the class and how the white students might feel if they were an only white person in a situation.

And then there was the time when a white student reported removing black and white, stating, "black is pure evilness and white pure goodness." This brought forth an immediate angry reply from an African-American woman who said she was sick of such thinking—"devil's food cake is brown and fattening and angel food cake is white, light, airy, and not fattening; and there is black cat, black Sunday, black sheep, black magic, the Black Plague, and the rest." No matter that the white woman protested that *she* had not meant to be racist. No argument did anything but vividly show the whole class how deeply pervasive racism is in our culture and how our language maintains it.

THE GROUP

Constructivism, with its emphasis on context and multiple, socially determined meanings, suggests that the persons who come to a group–any group–come with their own particulars that make up their own realities, and they will each be different. For the group worker, apprehending the elusive meaning of the other(s)' life experiences with some degree of fidelity becomes *the* challenge–the stuff of observation, definition, and interpretation. The struggle for the worker is to grasp and connect with these differences, to do no violence to each individual's expressions, to help members understand each other's meanings, and to accept the cacophony that characterizes group work.

Regardless of what groups decide as their agenda, the content of group work is *always* the experience of the other(s). And because of this, groups are powerful. The power of the group is the power to define reality, and therefore the meaning of experience. In the small group literature, group force has been variously referred to as group-think, peer pressure, behavior contagion, or the push toward conformity. But the real power is the elusive obvious, the power to amplify and support some meanings and ignore or reject other meanings.

Thus, the group is known to be the ideal medium for consciousness-raising. It is an intimate and mutually supportive situation for discussion of lived traumas, for examination of the relationship between individual experience and political ascription, and for subsequent social action.

In the following excerpt, the group worker engages professional working women in consciousness-raising and social action:

> Ann said she didn't see much of a problem for females getting ahead, that her daughter is a lawyer. Debra said to her, "Yes. But how many female lawyers in our area are partners in law firms? And what cases do they give your daughter?" Ann said she hadn't thought about it that way before. Then Carol brought up a problem. While shopping at the Mall, she saw some T shirts showing a heart, a spade, and a club card with this inscription: "I ♥ my dog; I ♠ my cat; I ♣ my wife." The group members were quite upset about this and discussed possible courses of action. Ann said that before coming to this group she probably would not have thought about the significance of this statement. The group decided two members would go to the Mall and talk to the vendor. The rest would call. They also decided to tell other people outside the group to call and express their concern.

In the next piece of work, a white, middle-aged worker with a job corps program for low-income youth is meeting with the few females learning auto mechanics–five African American, one Puerto Rican, and one white. The group is working on ways to cope with sexual harassment by male students and potential employers. The worker is struck by her awareness of her difference from these women: difference in age, difference in language, and difference in cultural background. This is what she wrote:

> The scene they were role playing involved a female job corps student being approached by a male student in a disrespectful way and it was up to the female student to handle the situation in a diplomatic way. "Why you be sweating me?" Mary yelled. The male student, portrayed by Red, replied, "Hey, Girl, it ain't all about you!" I asked the group to interpret this interaction with me since I was unfamiliar with their slang. They laughed and told me that when a guy is in your face trying to flirt with you, he is *sweating you. It ain't all about you* is a typical male response to a female rejecting him. He believes that she is stuck on herself since she is not interested in him.

The worker asked the group to teach her what she needed to know at that moment. She has learned that she does not have to know everything.

The essence of constructivism is understanding that the meaning of an event is not in the event itself nor in the behavior of the behaving person. Rather, it is in the mind of the constructing observer. This makes interpretation precarious. Consider Gergen's example:

> "Her boss approached her with steady gaze and ready smile." How is the reader to interpret the line? What is the author's intent? For a teenage subcommunity obsessed with romance, the "steady gaze" and "ready smile" are the obvious signals of a budding love affair, so clearly the author intends to write about love. In contrast, a business executive might assume the author was describing a popular managerial style. If the reader were a feminist, however, the "steady gaze" and "ready smile" might reveal the nuances of sexual harassment. (1991, 104-105)

Doing sensitive group work has always involved taking seriously how difficult it is to connect with anyone else, let alone with a group of several other persons. Such a connection involves appreciating the disturbance that your presence inevitably injects into any encounter with others and realizing that you *must* interact subjective-ly, for you can neither be objective nor be unaffected by the other(s). Group work necessitates knowing/feeling your own vulnerability when facing a group. It also requires connecting with the specifics of your own life in order to avoid confusing your self with the selves of the group members.

Contextually aware group work requires discarding all generaliza-tions about different ethnicities–generalizations proposed to make one ethnic-sensitive. What such generalizations actually do is ob-scure the real and rich within-group differences, and provide a false sense of understanding other people's worlds and meanings. They operate much like the stereotypes they were intended to replace. Contextual practice requires *thick*, grounded understanding, a famil-iarity with the details and particulars of the lived and living situation of each person in the group. This is consistent with the postmodern emphasis on personal and local knowing, valuing the unique more than the general, multiple realities, and being sensitive to the cultural context of each group member. The serious worker starts from scratch with each person in each group, learning from all of them what they mean by what they say as they continue together.

In some public schools there are support groups for children whose parents are divorced. The only commonality among the chil-dren in such groups may be that they are children of divorce. The context in which each divorce occurred may have been quite differ-ent and the meaning to each child is its own thing. One child may be relieved that the fighting has ended. His home is peaceful now. Another may be delighted that she will no longer be battered nor sexually molested. Her home may feel safer now. One child may feel homeless because his parents have joint custody and he is shuttled between two homes. Another may feel bereft at the loss of the parent who left. Still another may be angry at the parent who abandoned him by leaving, or feel guilty that she was not good enough to keep her parents together. There may be myriad combinations and per-mutations of such felt realities as well, and the worker must do more than assume a common bond. The diversity must be expressed, appreciated, and validated. It is the worker's job to do this and, more important to help the children do this with each other.

The perspective on context is important not only for highlighting within-group differences, but also for appreciating and working in accord with between-group differences. For example, a worker in Martin County, Kentucky, who wanted to develop a support group for wives of coal miners who were on strike, spoke with different women in an effort to determine a convenient time and place for them to meet. In consideration of the hecticness of their life situations, they met at his aunt's house, after the Sunday church service and before the church services on Tuesday. His aunt's house was near the church. The purpose of the group was to help members cope with the difficulties of the strike and develop a support network to draw on each others strengths to make it through the strike. Group work texts do not suggest meeting in someone's house, let alone one's aunt's house. For this group in this circumstance the aunt's living room was just fine.

This is not to fault group work texts. They could not possibly provide all the local know-how for understanding all of the people and circumstances where group work is practiced. So, in addition to learning general guidelines for working with groups, the group worker in his aunt's living room had to prepare like an anthropologist, immersing himself in the local knowledge that made up the context of his work, and in the personal stories that are the lives of the people. Then he had to think like a deconstructionist, asking himself what was not being said? who was not talking? And he needed to seek out and listen to the marginalized voices and center them in his attention: in this instance the wives of the striking miners.

IMPLICATIONS FOR PRACTICE

A constructivist mindset has been proposed as a way of looking at one's group work. Such a mentality becomes a special lens through which the worker views her practice, a lens that magnifies her context and that of every group participant. Thus, apprehending the others' meanings is the stuff of observation, definition, and interpretation. It is a thinking act that starts with first plans for the group and continues throughout the life of the work. It precedes whatever action the worker takes. But it is not the stuff of action. Constructivist thinking does not tell the worker what to do. And yet, everything the worker does is conditioned by how she thinks about what she will do. What the worker does will come from whatever theory of group work she holds, from the principles she has learned and follows for guiding her practice, from her own rich life experience, and from the value base and the professional code of ethics that the social worker follows.

According to constructivist thinking, one is not and cannot be the expert on another's situation. This is a humbling realization. It allows room for intuitive and tacit knowings and eliminates the pretense of objectivity. For social work practice is subjective and the worker is part of the work.

Constructivism necessitates attending consciously and skeptically to matters of perception. One must "look with planned emptiness," that is, cultivate an area in one's mind that is reserved for the unknown–an empty cell in one's frame of reference to reduce the likelihood that one will not see something because it is not in one's own experience (Middleman and Goldberg Wood, 1990, 24).

Constructivism also suggests that inferences are suspect. Each one needs to be checked out in order to find out if one is on the right track. It suggests that one should look and listen a lot and be suspicious when the main voice one hears is one's own. It is up to the worker to leave room for others' meanings to be expressed and to help this happen. The worker need not, and in fact cannot, solve the group's problems–quite a relief, although deflating, perhaps, when taken seriously.

Clearly, contextual group work requires an embrace of space–a place for all members to flex their thoughts, stretch their minds to accommodate new meanings, and bend their biases and notions of what is and should be in new directions.

REFERENCES

Berger, P. & Luckmin, T. (1967). *The Social Construction of Reality.* London: Penguin.

Bilides, D. (1990). Race, Color, Ethnicity and Class: Issues of Biculturalism in School-based Adolescent Counseling Groups, *Social Work with Groups*, 13:4, 43-58.

Brinkley, A. (1993). The 43% President, *Courier Journal.* Louisville, KY. July 11.

Brown, R. (1992). Poetics, Politics, and Truth: An Invitation to Rhetorical Analysis, in R. Brown (ed.), *Writing the Social Text.* New York: Aldine de Gruyer.

Bruner, J. (1986). Actual Minds, Possible Worlds. Cambridge, MA: Harvard University Press.

Chambers, C. (1992). Uphill All the Way: Reflections on the Course and Study of Welfare History, *Social Service Review,* 66:4, 492-504.

Chau, K. (1990). Facilitating Bicultural Development and Intercultural Skills in Ethnically Heterogeneous Groups, *Social Work with Groups,* 13:4, 1-5.

DeAnda, D. (1984). Bicultural Socialization: Factors Affecting the Minority Experience, *Social Work,* 25:2, 101-107.

Garland, J. (1992). From the Chairperson's Pen: In Defense of the Longer Group, *Social Work with Groups Newsletter,* 8:2, 1-2.

Geertz, C. (1983). *Local Knowledge.* New York: Basic Books.

Gergen, K. (1991). *The Saturated Self.* New York: Basic Books.

Goldberg, G. & Middleman, R. (1980). It Might Be a Boa Constrictor Digesting an Elephant: Vision Stretching in Social Work Education, *International Journal of Contemporary Social Work Education,* 3:1, 213-225.

Goldstein, H. (1990). Strength or Pathology: Ethical and Rhetorical Contrasts in Approaches, *Families in Society,* 71:5, 267-275.

Goodman, N. (1984). *Of Mind and Other Matters.* Cambridge, MA: Harvard University Press.

Guba, E. & Lincoln, Y. (1989). *Fourth Generation Evaluation.* Newbury Park, CA: Sage.

Hoffman, L. (1990). Constructing Realities: An Art of Lenses, *Family Process,* 29:1, 1-12.

Laird, J. (1989). Women and Stories: Restoring Women's Self-Constructions, in M. McGoldrick, C. Anderson & F. Walsh (eds.), *Women in Families.* New York: Norton, 422-450.

Lewis, E. (1992). Regaining Promise: Feminist Perspectives for Social Group Work Practice, *Social Work with Groups,* 15:2/3, 271-284.

Lukes, C. & Land, H. (1990). Biculturality and Homosexuality, *Social Work,* 35:2, 155-161.

Middleman, R. (1985). Perception and Cognition as Resources for Change. In D. Waldfogel & A. Rosenblatt (eds.), *Handbook of Clinical Practice.* San Francisco: Jossey-Bass.

Middleman, R. & Goldberg Wood, G. (1993). So Much for the Bell Curve: Constructionism, Power/Conflict and the Structural Approach to Direct Practice in Social Work, *Journal of Teaching in Social Work,* 8:1/2, 129-146.

_____ . (1991). Seeing/Believing/Seeing, *Social Work,* 36:3, 243-246.

_____ . (1990). *Skills for Direct Practice in Social Work.* New York: Columbia University Press.

_____ . (1985). Maybe It's a Priest or a Lady with a Hat with a Tree on It. Or Is It a Bumble Bee? Teaching Group Workers to See. *Social Work with Groups,* 8:1, 3-15.

Strom, K. & Gingerich, W. (1993). Educating Students for the New Market Realities, *Journal of Social Work Education,* 29:1, 78-87.

Swigonski, M. (1993). Feminist Standpoint Theory and the Questions of Social Research, *Affilia*, 8:2, 171-183.

Van Den Bergh, N. (1990). Managing Biculturalism at the Workplace: A Group Approach, *Social Work with Groups*, 13:4, 71-84.

von Glasersfeld, E. (1984). An Introduction to Radical Constructivism, in P. Watzlawick (ed.), *The Invented Reality*. New York: Norton, 17-40.

Weick, A. (1991). The Place of Science in Social Work, *Sociology and Social Welfare*, 18:4, 13-33.

Chapter 2

Uncovering Latent Content in Groups

Sondra Brandler
Camille P. Roman

There was a table set out under a tree in front of the house, and the March Hare and the Hatter were having tea at it: a Dormouse was sitting between them, fast asleep, and the other two were using it as a cushion, resting their elbows on it, and talking over its head. "Very uncomfortable for the Dormouse," thought Alice; "only as it's asleep, I suppose it doesn't mind."

The table was a large one, but the three were all crowded together at one corner of it. "No room! No room!" they cried out when they saw Alice coming. "There's plenty of room!" said Alice indignantly, and she sat down in a large armchair at one end of the table.

"Have some wine," the March Hare said in an encouraging tone. Alice looked all around the table, but there was nothing on it but tea. "I don't see any wine,"she remarked.

"There isn't any," said the March Hare.

"Then it wasn't very civil of you to offer it," said Alice angrily.

"It wasn't very civil of you to sit down without being invited," said the March Hare.

"I didn't know it was your table," said Alice: "it's laid for a great many more than three."

"Your hair wants cutting," said the Hatter. He had been looking at Alice for some time with great curiosity, and this was his first speech.

Special thanks to Sara Mitchell for her contribution to this article.

"You should learn not to make personal remarks," Alice said with some severity. "It's very rude."

The Hatter opened his eyes very wide on hearing this; but all he said was, "Why is a raven like a writing desk?"

Come, we shall have some fun now! thought Alice. I'm glad they've begun asking riddles–"I believe I can guess that," she added aloud.

"Do you mean that you think you can find out the answer to it?" said the March Hare.

"Exactly so," said Alice.

"Then you should say what you mean," the March Hare went on.

"I do," Alice hastily replied; "at least–at least I mean what I say–that's the same thing, you know."

"Not the same thing a bit!" said the Hatter. "Why, you might just as well say that 'I see what I eat' is the same thing as 'I eat what I see'!"

"You might just as well say," added the March Hare, "that 'I like what I get' is the same thing as 'I get what I like'!"

"You might just as well say," added the Dormouse, which seemed to be talking in its sleep, "that 'I breathe when I sleep' is the same thing as 'I sleep when I breathe'!"

"It is the same thing with you," said the Hatter, and here the conversation dropped, and the party sat silent for a minute, while Alice thought over all she could remember about ravens and writing desks, which wasn't much.

The Hatter was the first to break the silence. "What day of the month is it?" he said, turning to Alice: he had taken his watch out of his pocket, and was looking at it uneasily, shaking it every now and then, and holding it to his ear.

Alice considered a little, and then said, "The fourth."

"Two days wrong!" sighed the Hatter. "I told you butter wouldn't suit the works!" he added, looking angrily at the March Hare.

"It was the best butter," the March Hare angrily replied.

"Yes, but some crumbs must have got in as well," the Hatter grumbled: "you shouldn't have put it in with the bread knife."

The March hare took the watch and looked at it gloomily: then he dipped it into his cup of tea, and looked at it again: but he could think of nothing better to say than his first remark, "It was the best butter, you know."

Alice had been looking over his shoulder with some curiosity. "What a funny watch!" she remarked. "It tells the day of the month and doesn't tell what o'clock it is!"

"Why should it?" muttered the Hatter. "Does your watch tell you what year it is?"

"Of course not," Alice replied very readily: "but that's because it stays the same year for such a long time together."

"Which is just the case with mine," said the Hatter.

Alice felt dreadfully puzzled. The Hatter's remark seemed to her to have no sort of meaning in it, and yet it was certainly English. "I don't quite understand you," she said, as politely as she could.

"The Dormouse is asleep again," said the Hatter, and he poured a little hot tea upon its nose.

The Dormouse shook its head impatiently, and said, without opening its eyes, "Of course, of course: just what I was going to remark myself."

"Have you guessed the riddle yet?" the Hatter said, turning to Alice again.

"No, I give it up," Alice replied. "What's the answer?"

"I haven't the slightest idea," said the Hatter.

"Nor I," said the March Hare.

Alice sighed wearily, "I think you might do something better with the time," she said, "than wasting it in asking riddles that have no answers."

–Lewis Carroll
Alice's Adventures in Wonderland

The notion that unconscious motivations underlie all human encounters is a basic principle of psychotherapy and a cornerstone of individual treatment. In groups, too, another level of meaning exists below the surface. What is initially apparent is not necessarily what is really going on; what is seen and heard may be a symbolic way of saying something else or something more. Every comment, even if taken at face value, can have a myriad of meanings. The madcap antics in the preceding piece from *Alice's Adventures in Wonderland*, although a satiric fantasy, focus on the different ways in which we understand communication. The March Hare's table appears to have plenty of room for guests yet the party goers all assure Alice that there is no room at all. What is the real meaning here? Is it that there really is no room at the table or is it that the other guests are unable to make room for her? The wine that Alice is offered is actually nonexistent. What is being offered then? Is it the Hare's concept of wine or is it nothing at all?

The excerpt is rich in examples related to the complexity of communication, but in real life as well, the interpretations of what is really meant and their relation to what is said are as varied as every speaker and every listener. The speaker may believe he wants to communicate one idea but, through body language, tone, and word choice, may actually communicate something else. The failure to communicate an accurate message may lie in unconscious motivations. These motivations lead to communicating thoughts not consciously intended or to selective hearing, also the result of unconscious feelings, by those addressed. In groups, communication is complicated by the many different speakers and respondents and the psychological baggage which each brings to the group setting. The fact that, in groups, we deal with numerous people at the same time makes transferences and countertransferences more complex (Yalom, 1985).

The group has its own personality derived from the individual personalities of its members interacting as each struggles with conflicting feelings. The group is greater than the sum of its parts because there is a seemingly infinite number of interrelationships among the members creating different wholes. There are both a group consciousness (a shared understanding motivated by latent dynamics) and many individual consciousness each with its own latent qualities.

The nature of the latent material is strongly influenced by the needs of the group members and the group phase. In order to proceed further with this discussion, a brief review of phase theory might be helpful. Throughout the lifetime of the group, and indeed through the lifetime of each session, the group moves from a beginning phase of introduction of the work, to a middle phase of struggle with the group tasks and content, and finally to a termination phase of separating from the group and moving on to other challenges (Garland, Kolodny, and Jones, 1975). Each of these phases is characterized by specific tasks for group members and for the worker.

The beginning phase is generally the first third of the group's life. It is essentially an orientation stage that involves certain issues, including the development of trust and the overcoming of mistrust in a new and unknown environment. It is a time of tuning-in, testing, and watching, approaching the desired acceptance, and avoiding the feared rejection. It is a time of struggle to identify and define expectations for oneself and for others. It is a time to develop a way of being in a group, which defines the norms and establishes some roles. There is a need to identify the purposes that have brought members together and how the group will address those purposes, all of which lead to the establishment of a working contract. Beginnings are a time of great promise and yet a time of considerable trepidation.

The middle phase, generally known as the work phase, constitutes the second third of the group's life. The middle phase may be divided further to include an early middle phase, in which the major issues of trust are resolved sufficiently to permit the work to take place. The work of middles involves the movement toward the development of intimacy, allowing risk-taking, confrontation, and problem-solving, and the engagement and resolution of conflicts. The level of safety and cohesiveness permits members in this phase to expose more of themselves and to try on new roles. Middles is an exciting and vibrant period, one of growth and challenge.

The final phase, termination, generally the last part of the group's life, occurs in small measure earlier on in the end of each meeting, in the departure of a member or worker, and in the movement from one phase to another. A powerful and underaddressed phase, it is characterized by loss and separation felt acutely by worker and group members. Here there is a need to identify and consolidate gains to help members go forth, even though they mourn the loss of the group and its safety. In termination, group members begin to recognize their accomplishments as separate from those of the group, allowing each member to go forward to establish new and productive relationships. It is a time to mourn what members hoped to do and could not, a time of regrets and hope.

Throughout the course of the group, the worker, in whatever phase, has the difficult task of uncovering the latent issues of the group personality and individual members' personalities so as to propel the group forward toward resolving conflict and maximizing mutual work leading to growth. If not addressed, the latent themes will haunt the group and block its ability to achieve its goals. The process of reaching for latent content involves a new kind of listening, new in its capacity for hearing what is left unsaid and for ferreting out the connections between what occurs on the surface and what may be happening below (Garvin, 1974).

THE USE OF SELF

What we have said so far about latent content concerns the group and its members without regard to the unconscious or latent factors which motivate the worker. The worker, after all, is no more a tabula rasa than are her group members. Ideally, what keeps her on track is the conscious way in which she constantly monitors her own reactions and listens for feedback. One hopes the goals of the group have been developed after reviewing the needs of the population, the clients' expressed goals for the group experience, and the needs and goals of the agency. Each session, the worker contemplates general and specific goals to assist the group. The worker's determinations about areas for work will be connected to her knowledge about the goals for the group in any particular session as well as over the lifetime of the group.

The worker may not set up the group agenda to deal with what she deems important; rather she will listen for the content which reveals what is important to the group goals and to her knowledge of the population. If certain areas key to the needs of the population seem to be addressed only peripherally or avoided altogether, the worker may infer that some resistance is present. Some of this resistance may be accentuated by the worker's own difficulty with the material.

A worker in a mastectomy group, for example, knows that issues concerning body image and sexuality need to be explored if the overall goal of the group (adjustment to the crisis of a breast amputation) is to be achieved. In early group meetings, these issues are unlikely to be addressed; resistance to such discussion is probable. Such matters involve intimate self-disclosure and are difficult for many people to talk about, particularly in a beginning phase. Though these issues may continue to be unaddressed, nevertheless they are present, part of the latent material, and probably problematic on some level because they get in the way of the group's work.

The reasons these or other issues remain submerged may have to do not only with their delicacy but with the message the worker gives that she, too, finds the discussion uncomfortable; the worker's own issues of loss and sexual identity are triggered in even a benign comment alluding to sexuality. She squirms, moves the content elsewhere, picks up on another issue. The latent message she communicates, that this is too frightening to talk about, threatens the ability of the group to explore painful issues.

Clues to latent content are found throughout each session. Body language, an unexplained feeling of tension in the room, sadness, anger, a tone that seems inappropriate to affect, affect that seems inappropriate to content, a repeated avoidance of emotionally charged material, and many intangibles alert the worker to another level of meaning. Although she can never be certain what is going on, the worker needs to be sensitive to her own feelings, willing to pursue those about which she is unclear. She may ask directly about the feeling she is experiencing or a pattern she is observing: "Everybody seems so quiet today. What's going on?" Or she may offer a tentative interpretation: "It seems every time people start to talk about how scared they feel, someone changes the topic. I wonder what that's about." Group members may continue to claim that nothing special is happening. Perhaps they are not ready to confront troubling subjects; perhaps they are still unaware of other things they are feeling. Ongoing querying, exploring, and striving to understand the symbolic ways in which communication is proceeding all help the group to reach its goals. If the worker models a method of meaningful exploration, group members learn how to participate in the process.

We have developed a useful tool to help the worker identify latent content in any particular session (Roman, 1980), and we will illustrate the use of the tool by examining a process excerpt taken from an actual group session.

The group from which this piece of process is excerpted is a newsletter group for adolescents. The purposes of the group include: to produce a newsletter that is distributed to various settlement house sites; to address developmental tasks of adolescence, including identity formation and gender issues, self-esteem building, mastery of specific skills, development of positive peer relationships, separation and individuation issues, and cooperative work skills; and to encourage creative expression (Schaffer and Pollak, 1987).

There are five teenagers participating in the following session. Yolanda is a 15-year-old of Puerto Rican descent who has been a highly verbal member of the group for over a year. She lives with her mother and two younger brothers. Ellen is a 16-year-old of African-American descent who has been an active member of the group for several years. She lives with her parents and older and younger sisters. Ed is a 15-year-old Dominican who has been living in the United States for three years. He joined the group in the later sessions of the past year and has only recently begun to participate. He lives with his mother, 17-year-old brother, and three younger sisters. Cindy is a 14-year-old Caucasian who is of Polish descent. She has been in the group less than a year and tends to comment infrequently but with some sarcasm. She lives with her mother. Keisha is a 15-year-old Jamaican who recently relocated to the United States with her father and stepmother. She is attending the group for the first time. The worker, Sharon, is a 23-year-old Caucasian of Irish descent. She is a graduate social work student who has had some volunteer experience working with children.

The newsletter group runs during the school year from September to June. The vignette is from the first meeting of a new season with a new student intern. The worker has been informed by her predecessor that the last edition of the newsletter has not been printed because of a controversy over a fictional story written by Ellen, one of the group members. The story is a highly explicit, stark, and powerful commentary on teenage sexuality, misogyny, and the possible consequences of unprotected sex–pregnancy and HIV transmission. Fearing the negative repercussions on funding of printing such a story, the executive director of the agency has held up production of the newsletter.

A few minutes into the session, Ellen begins to hint at how upset she is over the failure of the agency to publish her story. The worker picks up on Ellen's clues and responds by saying, "I wonder if Ellen is feeling a little like she doesn't want to get involved in the group this year–I mean why bother if you're not sure what you write will be published, huh?" Ellen is receptive to this intervention and begins to express her feelings of frustration over the story, stating that she does not know what they want from her and that what she writes about is real. The other teens join the discussion in support of Ellen. For several minutes, there is a general discussion about how boys are disrespectful toward girls.

Yolanda: What you wrote about is really real. I know a lot of boys that say "I bagged this girl" or "I got that one last night." They're really nasty sometimes.

Ed: Yeah, guys are always talking crazy-like. They say "Man, I had this girl and her leg was all up by her ear," or "Oh yeah, well this honey I was with, I had her wrapped up like a pretzel."

Ellen: I know. The boys I hang out with are always talking like that, but they don't want me to write about what really goes on.

Cindy: No, but it's the truth. What should we write about? Fairy tales and butterflies?

Worker: So, you all are saying that you can really understand Ellen's story. This is stuff you deal with all the time.

Keisha: You know, I hear a lot of boys near my house who talk just like that or who make bets about how many girls they can be with. It's just a game for them. Guys always be dissing on girls.

Ed: Naw, not all of them. I know guys who really like girls, but they won't even look their way.

Yolanda: No. Boys are just trying to be cool with their friends and try to show off by saying "Yeah, I been with her. She's good," or "Aah, I can't believe you did that ugly girl! You can't get nobody better than that?"

Ed: Not every boy. Some of them, yeah.

Worker: So, Ed, you're saying that maybe different people experience this issue in a different way. Your experience is that not all boys act this way?

Ed: Yeah, not every guy's like that.

Ellen: No, but most of them are. I hear boys talk about girls all the time, just like in my story.

Worker: You know, how this relates to the newsletter group may be in learning to think how our readers will take what we write about. In Ellen's story, she means to let everyone know that if you mess around you might get hurt, like get pregnant or get AIDS, but what if someone reads the story and thinks that Ellen meant only to say all boys are dogs, even though Ed said they aren't? What if someone doesn't understand what Ellen meant to say? One thing that we'll learn in doing the newsletter is how to be responsible for the kinds of messages we may be giving our readers. Well, maybe we should talk about what we want to do in the newsletter group this year. Let's try to come up with some ideas about how we would like the newsletter to be.

In this excerpt, latent themes are present which the worker may or may not have identified. By charting certain variables, worker's feelings, members' feelings, population dynamics, group phase issues, and manifest content, the worker can make some educated guesses about what is happening. The worker can easily connect variables in the chart with her knowledge about the population and the phase. The chart demands the worker's acknowledgement of her own feelings in the process, which is necessary to a clearer understanding of her interventions or her difficulty in intervening. The chart, with some suggested entries, is included as Figure 2.1.

To use the chart to identify the latent themes, the worker first must look at the manifest content, what is actually talked about in the meeting. In this excerpt, the group is clearly focused on the fact that an article submitted to the newsletter was not published. They also generally discuss male/female relationships and some of the stereotypes members have regarding the opposite sex. By tracking these manifest themes across the various categories, the worker begins to see connections. Some of the manifest issues related to the article publication can be identified in other categories. For the purpose of illustration, we will only track one of the manifest content entries: the story not being approved for publication.

The worker may look first to material in the column on population dynamics. It is immediately apparent that the issue of publication suggests adolescent issues regarding identity formation (this is who we are and what we are about), establishment of independence, and separation and individuation (Blos, 1962). By examining the column I labeled "group phase issues," the worker sees that this same manifest content appears also to reflect beginning phase issues of trust/mistrust (can members trust that the worker will respect them and recognize their needs).

In addition, the beginning issues of expectations are being explored. What can the members expect that the worker will do regarding the publication of the story and, in turn, regarding every aspect of the group? Ally with them? Protect them? Demand of them? Challenge them? Accept them? Reject them? The testing and introduction of self characteristic of the beginning phase, also relates to the content of the unpublished story (a story of highly explicit, stark, and powerful commentary on teenage sexuality, misogyny, and the possible consequences of unprotected sex). The particular introduction of the only male member of the group, Ed, reflects his need to differentiate himself from other boys–those who take advantage of girls–again a part of members' struggles with the approach/avoidance characteristic of beginnings.

Having identified the relationships between one part of the manifest content, the developmental tasks of adolescents, and the beginning phase issues, the worker can draw her attention to those important affective components. The worker's feelings also relate to the unpublished story. She is afraid of being rejected. She needs the group's acceptance and recognizes that she is viewed as a representative of the agency which has refused publication. This concern connects to her feelings of role confusion. Is she the authority, the representative of the agency, or is she an advocate for the teenagers? Is she a young person like the adolescents or an authority figure who will be separate from them?

When the worker examines the column of the chart describing members' feelings, she can observe some conflicts the adolescents experience which are similar to those of her own. Both worker and

FIGURE 2.1

Worker's Feelings	Members' Feelings	Population Dynamics	Group Phase Issues	Manifest Content	Latent Content
Confusion with her role as authority	*Fear of rejection*	**Developmental**	*Trust/Mistrust*	*Story not being approved for publication*	*The beginning issue of trust and mistrust parallels the adolescent developmental issues of identity formation and separation and individuation*
Need to be accepted by group	*Need to be accepted*	*Identity formation*	*Approach/Avoidance*		
	Mistrust of worker and agency	Development of self-esteem	*Expectations of a) Workers b) Members*	Relationship between males and females	
Fear of rejection	Mistrust of peer group	Mastery of specific skills	Beginning development of norms, goals, and contract		
Confusion re: purpose of group (task or therapy)	*Disrespect from members, worker, and agency*	Development of peer relationships	*Introduction of self*	Stereotypes	
		Separation/Individuation	High level dependency on worker		
Fear of being incompetent	*Feeling misunderstood by members, authority*	*Dependence/Independence*	Beginning development of cohesiveness		
	Feeling angry	**Socioeconomic and Cultural:**	Role development a) Worker b) Members		
		Learned dependency and powerlessness			
		Racism contributing to low self-esteem and negative self-image			
		Stigmatized population a) Gender b) Class			
		Cultural differences regarding the group's sexual norms, roles, values, and issues of authority			

(note: Italicized factors are interconnected to derive latent themes) members have feelings about rejection and acceptance expressed in the manifest content of the publication being accepted or rejected. Members also express issues around mistrust directed toward the worker because she is an agency representative and toward other members of the group who they do not yet really know. Some of the suspiciousness about the process of rejecting the story leads group members to be angry. In fact, the anger is an undercurrent in many of the adolescents' expressed feelings.

We have chosen one piece of the manifest content to follow in various columns of the chart, but any of the pieces can be explored in a similar fashion to further uncover latent themes. The worker can conclude from this analysis that one latent theme in this vignette concerns the beginning issue of trust and mistrust paralleled with the adolescent developmental issues of identity formation, and separation and individuation. Once a worker has identified patterns and the interrelationships among the entries in the various columns of the chart, she can begin to choose areas for focus, addressing issues from any arena in which she feels comfortable. Knowledge of the latent content does not necessitate immediate intervention around these themes. The worker's awareness of latent issues simply guides her approach and suggests avenues for exploration.

The chart can be used at various stages in a worker's professional development. For the beginning worker, who often struggles with the integration of cognitive material and her own feelings in an effort to make effective interventions, it provides a way to reflect after a group session and to prepare for the next. For the seasoned worker, who may be struggling to decipher a particularly confusing interaction, perhaps because of her own countertransferential issues, the chart helps her to step back and objectively evaluate the situation.

The latent content is a vital part of the group process. Without recognizing and addressing it, we remain on a superficial level and the group is prevented from achieving its goals.

REFERENCES

Blos, Peter (1962). *On Adolescence: A Psychoanalytic Interpretation*, New York: The Free Press.

Brandler, Sondra and Roman, Camille P. (1991). *Group Work: Skills and Strategies for Effective Interventions*, New York: The Haworth Press, Inc.[1]

Garland, James, Kolodny, Ralph and Jones, Hubert (1975). "A Model for Stages of Development in Social Work Groups," *Explorations in Group Work*, Saul Bernstein, ed., Boston: Milford House, Inc., pp. 17-71.

Garvin, Charles D. (1974). "Group Process: Usages and Uses in Social Work Practice," *Individual Change Through Small Groups,* Glaser, Paul, Sarri, Rosemary, and Vinter, Robert, eds., New York: Free Press, pp. 209-233.

Roman, Camille (1980). "Group Processing Chart," Mimeo.

Schaffer, Stephen and Pollak, Jerrold (1987). "Listening to the Adolescent Therapy Group," *Group, The Journal of the Eastern Group Psychotherapy Society*, 11(3), pp. 155-164.

Yalom, I (1985). "The Therapist Transference and Transparency," *The Theory and Practice of Group Psychotherapy*, 3rd ed., New York: Basic Books.

---

[1]Portions of this text have been excerpted for use in this paper.

Chapter 3

Social Group Work Competence: Our Strengths and Challenges

Maeda J. Galinsky
Janice H. Schopler

We welcome this opportunity to join with you to celebrate our strengths and consider the challenges we face as social group workers. There have been times in our past when group services seemed to be on the wane and when we were worried about our identity as social group workers, but this is not our current concern. As the papers and workshops at this symposium illustrate, groups are being used to respond to a vast array of individual and societal needs, problems, and issues. We are reaching out to new populations and to populations we have served in the past–the homeless, people with HIV-related disease, the violent and their victims, immigrants, the frail elderly and their families, children in need, angry adolescents, and the mentally ill. Groups are widely viewed as an important method not just for educating, supporting, socializing, and treating individuals, but also for empowering people and creating social change. In past decades, we were often hard-pressed to find any mention of groups, but now groups are a part of our culture. We have a high profile and get lots of attention, even in the popular press. The growing popularity of groups became clear to us from the frequency with which groups are presented in one small facet of the media–the cartoon pages.

Plenary Address presented at the Fifteenth Annual Symposium of the Association for the Advancement of Social Work with Groups, New York City, New York, October 23, 1993.

Obviously, the public values groups and often assumes that any social worker can handle a group. The opportunities and the problems that come with the emergence of an increasingly complex society and the growing acceptance of social services have created an unprecedented demand for group work expertise. As social group work professionals, we have the compassion, the creativity, and the responsibility to respond to this demand, but do we have the competence? In this current "results-oriented" era, competence is the bottom line.

We will be using the concept of competence as a framework to identify our strengths–what we are doing well–and to identify our challenges–what we need to improve. We know of no panaceas and have no pronouncements to make about how group work can cure our troubled society. What we will be sharing with you is a report card, a measure of our current competence as social group workers. In the style of our esteemed president and first lady, this group work report card is based on our assessment of group work's past and future. As with all report cards, our judgment has a certain element of subjectivity. We do not necessarily expect you to agree with our assessment of group work, but we do hope we stimulate your thinking.

ASSESSING OUR COMPETENCE

We define competence as the ability to be responsive to the differential needs of diverse populations by drawing on existing resources and methods, and by developing new approaches. Our ability to be responsive as group workers derives from our theoretical and value base, our practice skills, and our research. Each of these components of group work competence are interdependent yet make a unique contribution to our ability to respond to the current and emerging needs of individuals and society. Our values define the direction and scope of practice, while our theoretical frameworks contribute conceptual guidance for practice, and research. Our practice methods, skills, and techniques are the core of our competence. They may be theoretically grounded and empirically tested, or they may be the intuitive, caring responses that are born from practice wisdom, necessity, and the creativity of practitioners who care. Our research tests and expands our theoretical base, helps us refine our practice, and monitors our accountability and effectiveness.

To judge our competence as group workers, we shall examine the current status of group work theory and values, practice, and research, and grade the adequacy of our performance in each of these areas. Then we shall focus on what we need to do to improve. We hope our assessment will help us affirm our strengths and begin to address our challenges.

Our Theoretical and Value Base

As social group workers, we draw on an almost bewildering array of theoretical frameworks, models, and concepts to deal with the diversity of demands that face us. In an earlier era, we could organize our thinking around the three contrasting, yet complementary, models: the reciprocal, remedial, and social goals. In more recent years, these basic frameworks have grown with a virtual explosion of perspectives, including, but not limited to, cognitive behavioral, interactionist, humanistic, socio-educational, psycho-educational, growth, mainstream, task-centered, and empowerment approaches. We have analytic models that guide our planning and evaluation of group practice and we have process models that focus on the interplay among social workers members, and the group's environment. We have drawn on concepts from gestalt, guided group interaction, group psychotherapy, community organization, psychodrama, and learning theory, among others. We have concepts related to composition, goal setting, group development, programming, and ending. Certainly, for "breadth of perspective" we have earned top marks in group work theory! The heterogeneity of our theoretical frameworks is responsive to the multiple demands for our service.

We also share a core of values and concepts that give group work its unique identity and integrity as a social work method. Our diffuse perspectives are joined by common adherence to:

- Our trifocal view of three levels of intervention–individual, group, and environment
- Our humanistic values and responsiveness to societal issues and individual needs
- Our valuing of diversity and personal empowerment

- Our conceptualization of mutual aid
- Our programming concepts for structuring our work with groups

We have a rich heritage and common commitments to guide us as we continue to expand our theoretical frameworks. For this, we receive high marks. In general, social group work theory and values support a holistic approach and a reality focus. Our belief in the healing power of the group, captured in our concept of "mutual aid," has now been widely adopted and is an underlying principle of both the self-help and support group movements. Our attention to the environment enhances the power of our group interventions and serves as a deterrent to "blaming the victim."

Although our theoretical performance is exceptional in some areas, in others we note a need for improvement, namely: (1) general frameworks do not always apply to specific situations; (2) our transmission of group work theory and values is uneven; and (3) theoretical frameworks designed for face-to-face groups may provide only limited guidance for the groups created by technological advances. We need to address each of these areas to raise our grade in theory.

First, our conceptualization of group processes and principles tends to be general in nature, but we have not identified the caveats. Democratic procedures may, for example, be accepted by groups that come together voluntarily to solve common problems, but may be viewed with distrust by involuntary members who are attending a group by court order unless developed in the context of an empowerment approach. Group participation in formulating goals may be short-circuited by a time limit. We value difference and direct our interventions toward achieving cultural competence and an affirmation of diversity, acknowledging the importance of race, ethnicity, gender, and sexual orientation. We have not, however, developed the specific guidelines needed to ensure that our practice will be consistently responsive and respectful of differences. We need to reexamine our generalist guidelines and overarching values to define the boundaries, identify the exceptions, and operationalize the interventions that are necessary to implement critical concepts in specific situations.

Second, we have no assurance that social group work theory and values are being transmitted to all social workers, yet all social workers tend to be regarded as potential group leaders. Group work values and theories are an important, but not necessarily a required, part of the social work curriculum. Too often, group work theory is lost in a generalist curriculum or is not required at all, except in the field practicum. Yet, the general public, agency directors, and supervisors assume that social work students and practitioners "know about groups." When students and practitioners have not had an adequate grounding in group work theory and values, they turn to other group modalities for mentoring, guidance, and direction. This is a mixed blessing. We hope that they incorporate what they learn within the framework of social work, but there is no guarantee that they will discover on their own the values and principles that govern our practice.

Third, we have to expand our conception of groups. Our traditional concepts and values relate to face-to-face interactions among a worker and members. Technology has made that definition of groups obsolete. Groups can form and communicate by telephone and computer. At present, we have little theoretical guidance to give to leaders of these groups and have only begun to evaluate the adequacy of our current concepts in the light of new technology.

Our overall assessment of our competence in the area of theory and values indicates that we are lacking in some areas. Our theory provides general rather than specific guidance; we have not devel-. oped mechanisms for ensuring that all social workers know social group work theory and values; and we have not updated our theory to deal with new technology. With this in mind, we give social group work a high passing grade, but there remains plenty of room for improvement in regard to theory and values.

Our Practice

Our assessment of the current status of social group work practice is based on consultations with practitioners, our review of the group work literature, and what we have learned at this symposium and related meetings, such as the Empirical Foundations of Group Work Practice Symposium, the annual program meeting of CSWE, the annual conference of NASW, the ACOSA Symposium, the European Group Work Symposium, and more specialized conferences. The groups we have read about, heard about, and observed lead us to the conclusion that group work practice is flourishing. When past approaches prove ineffective, we are innovating and reaching out in new ways.

Our responsiveness is evident in our continued attention to the needs of children, youth, the elderly, and other dependent populations; in our attention to poverty, violence, and other social problems; in our concern for persons with AIDS, cancer, mental illness, and those who are suffering from other serious illnesses; in the support we provide immigrants, the unemployed, the bereaved, and others dealing with life transitions; and in our efforts to prevent unwanted pregnancy, provide job skills, promote more effective parenting, and offer opportunities for people to develop their potential. Our responsiveness is also evident in our outreach: groups are meeting in waiting rooms, churches, schools, health settings, shelters for the homeless and abused, clubhouse programs, and prisons. We are using new group forms and technology to make group services more accessible, as reflected in single-session groups, open-ended groups, telephone groups, and computer networks.

Technology has perhaps had more of an impact on group work than any other social work method. We are using audiovisual technology to educate group workers, to train practitioners, to provide group members with information, and to evaluate our effectiveness. We are beginning to use telephone conference lines to bring individuals with common conditions together to share their concerns, address their questions, and build supportive networks. We are beginning to see the development of computer networks that create groups that can respond to individual concerns and address societal problems at any hour of the day, as long as the net is "up" and operational.

The groups we organize, sponsor, and facilitate are characterized by attention to ethnicity, race, and culture, and are structured to provide opportunities for empowerment. They embody our recognition that people who come together with common problems and issues often have more to give to each other than we as workers can provide. As has been true throughout our history, group work practice is on the cutting edge and leads theory. Without a doubt, our practice meets the highest standards of competence.

We do, however, have two critical concerns about the current status of social group work practice. First, best practice too often is not replicated, and second, best practice at times loses out to concerns with efficiency. Some of our most creative and effective group interventions are never repeated because busy practitioners may not have the time to conceptualize and communicate their efforts and may not have the data to validate their outcomes. Because many social workers have no specialized training in group work, they may not have the theoretical base to develop their practice models and may be unfamiliar with the group work literature and networking opportunities such as this symposium. Our failure to capitalize on practice innovations represents lost opportunities.

Our practice competence is also constrained when organizational efficiency rather than concepts of best practice is the impetus for group formation. Practitioners who are directed to form groups so they can serve more clients and increase the agency census may not have adequate time for preparation and follow-up. They may have no training, supervision, or support for their work with groups. Groups formed under these conditions are at risk for negative outcomes for individual members, the group, and the organization. We support the efficient use of organizational and community resources, but groups should be designed and workers should be trained to respond to the needs of particular populations and not just to offer groups for the sake of efficiency.

We can take pride in our practice accomplishments, but we cannot rest on our laurels. We must renew our efforts to reach out and respond to individual and social needs with the best practice available. We must find ways to incorporate and refine practice innovations. We must also find ways to support practitioners. We have the concern and the commitment and a wealth of practice wisdom, but our superior grade in the area of practice will continue only if our practice efforts are undergirded by our development in the areas of theory and research.

Our Research

In an era of technological advances and complex societal problems, the credibility of our practice and the relevance of our theory rest on our research competence. Our assessment of our research competence is based on our examination of both qualitative and quantitative studies of group work practice and our review of practitioner efforts to evaluate group work practice. In this area, we commend our efforts as group workers. There has been a continuing increase in the amount of research literature available over the past several decades and in the emphasis given to the need for more systematic and rigorous research. However, we question the adequacy of our progress. Our review leads us to the following observations: (1) our research is still predominantly descriptive; (2) we do not evaluate our practice on a regular basis; and (3) we have not set a research agenda for social group work practice.

First, our review indicates that much of our group research is descriptive. Some of these descriptive studies are based on clearly defined concepts of intervention, process, and outcomes, and use fairly large samples for data collection. These studies provide a foundation for exploring research questions important to our development of theory and practice. Most often, however, our descriptive studies are based on the examination of a single group. Some systematic approach to data collection may be used, but the conclusions tend to rest on the subjective observation of the leader about group processes and outcomes. Although these practice descriptions can be helpful to practitioners who are working with similar populations and problems, they are limited for sake of generalization. They serve as exemplars of creative, responsive group practice, but do not address the relationship of interventions to the outcomes achieved. They fail to provide sufficient guidance for replicating and refining successful practice.

Second, as group workers we do not systematically evaluate our practice. Gaps in evaluation knowledge are the result of in a number of barriers. The time and money required for consistent evaluation of practice are scarce commodities in the lives of overworked and highly committed professionals. Although administrators want evidence of the effectiveness of group services, the tangible support needed for evaluation of practice may be limited. Available research designs utilizing control and comparison groups may be unrealistic given financial constraints and service imperatives. Standardized measures which capture the kinds of goals we pursue in our groups are often unavailable. Even given these constraints, however, there are opportunities missed to evaluate our practice with some degree of rigor.

Third, we are lacking a research agenda for social group work practice. In some respects, group work research is still in a formative stage, characterized by the independent examination of diffuse research questions. This reflects the richness of our practice but does not build a core of knowledge. We are beginning to define and measure group outcomes and identify some of the factors associated with positive and negative effects. We have identified critical group processes such as conflict resolution, mutual support, and group development, and we are studying how these processes affect outcomes. Unfortunately, we have little agreement on our operational definitions, use diverse methodologies, and seldom attempt to replicate results. Many of our studies do not move beyond the stage of exploratory research. We do not want to lose the energy and interest associated with differing approaches and independent exploration, but we cannot expand our knowledge about group outcomes, processes, and interventions unless we take account of what others have learned.

In summary, our research productivity is only moderate. Our assessment of our research competence indicates that we have learned a great deal over the years, but our research is formative in nature and our results are scattered. Too often, we do not use sufficient rigor to have valid and generalizable findings. Too often, we do not include a plan for evaluation in our group preparations. We must redouble our efforts to become more competent in the area of research.

OUR CHALLENGES

What then is our overall assessment of our group work competence? Our report card is one we can review with pride, but not complacency. Our broad theoretical base and humanistic values provide us with the necessary flexibility to be creative in responding to existing and emerging needs. Our practice is characterized by our responsiveness to individual and societal demands, by our willingness to use a range of approaches, by our commitment to empowerment of clients, and by our appreciation of diversity. We are beginning to evaluate our practice on a systematic basis and to refine our theory.

Our assessment of group work competence also indicates that we have some areas that need attention. Our performance in practice surpasses our theoretical and research accomplishments, yet our competence in any one area is linked to our competence in the other two areas. We cannot expand our practice capacity without adequate theoretical and research support. Our theoretical base cannot develop unless our ideas are tested in practice, and research. We cannot improve our research without recognizing the demands of practice and the limits of our theoretical base.

What are our challenges? We must pay more than lip service to the interdependent nature of group work theory, practice, and research. We must strive for group work competence by building on our strengths and taking action to overcome our limitations in each of these areas. We have shared our evaluation and now we offer our prescription for achieving true competence, a competence characterized by relevant theoretical frameworks, responsive services, and rigorous research.

ACHIEVING TRUE COMPETENCE

Relevant Theoretical Frameworks

The theoretical frameworks for group work must be reexamined in the light of our values to determine if they provide adequate guidance for practice and research. We know from our assessment of theoretical competence that our concepts need to be more explicitly defined. We must clearly identify desired outcomes for every group we serve. Potential negative experiences as well as positive ones must be identified. We must continue to examine the theoretical links between process and outcomes. Further, it is imperative that we begin to develop conceptual models for using new group forms, such as telephone and computer groups.

Our models must take specific account of multicultural issues, given the trends in our society. We must be prepared to adapt our models to the realities of current service, so that single-session, short-term, open-ended, and other evolving group forms are given the recognition and status they merit.

Responsive Service

To keep our service responsive, we must be proactive and ensure that our group service keeps pace with demand. We must be ready to consider new approaches to practice and to respond aggressively to social problems. We must listen to our clients and ensure that the methods we use provide them with opportunities for empowerment. We must be prepared to work at the individual or the environmental level. We must revise our practice as the results of evaluation research that give evidence of goals unachieved.

We need to reclaim our place in the social work curriculum and give increased attention to doctoral study of group work. We need to ensure that every social worker who leads a group has had some training for group work practice. We need further training in the use of new technologies, including telecommunications and computer networks.

Rigorous Research

As group work practitioners and educators, it is imperative that we find ways to overcome barriers to research. We must be able to demonstrate that the groups we serve reach effective outcomes. We must be ready to operationally define outcomes and develop measurement tools. As part of our research agenda, we need to ensure that every group leader has the skills and commitment necessary to evaluate group process and outcomes. We need to design rigorous tests of our practice to complement our exploratory studies of effectiveness.

We need to work to establish a research agenda as we cannot build a core of knowledge to test theory and guide practice without ongoing evaluation and controlled study. We must develop our research methodology, including design alternatives and user-friendly measures. We must advocate for research supports. We must develop models of collaborative research, with practitioners and researchers joining together in a partnership to build a more scientific basis for practice.

In conclusion, our challenges excite us with the promise of change. To improve our competence, we must study and conceptualize our current practice, we must capture and replicate "best practice," and we must publish our results. Our competence rests on our ability to develop our theory and transmit knowledge, to be responsive to the demands for group work services, and to demonstrate what we have accomplished. We celebrate with you our strengths as social group workers and we look forward to working on the challenges we face. Together we can make an important contribution to meeting the needs of our troubled society.

Chapter 4

Group Process in Administration Revisited

Joan C. Weiss
Paul H. Ephross

INTRODUCTION

Group work began with the realization that there are structures and processes that are common to all groups of all types. With its beginnings in group services agencies, it took half a century before group work permeated the entire field of social work and became an integral part of a large proportion of treatment programs. Throughout its development, an essential ingredient of group work theory and practice was its focus on the similarities of structure and process that characterize all types of groups and on the similarities and differences of skills needed for effective professional influence on the various types of groups.

Over the past half century or more, group work skills have been perceived as relevant to work with a progressively broader spectrum of types of clients, such as gang members, patients in residential settings, incarcerated offenders, relatives of patients with terminal illness, victims of ethnoviolence or other crimes, persons facing particular life crises, psychiatric in- and out-patients, couples under stress, and many others. Simultaneously, administrators and practitioners alike have realized that these skills can be useful for work with staff members in groups that cover the entire gamut of supervisory, administrative, and planning processes.

During the 1970s, the boundaries of group work as a field became unclear. One of the by-products of the splintering of group work into various functional fields has been a loss of focus on the entire spectrum of types of groups. As the validity and utility of social work with groups has been rediscovered, it has become apparent that administrative groups deserve renewed attention (Ephross, 1981; Toseland and Ephross, 1987; Ephross and Vassil, 1988, 1993). It is a positive development that recent textbooks on group work practice in general devote at least some focused attention to what have variously been called "task," or "working," or "administrative" groups (Toseland and Rivas, 1984; Garvin, 1987; Brown, 1991).

Social workers in all settings spend some of their professional time as members, chairs, or leaders of administrative groups. Typical examples are staff and committee meetings. Because most client problems that social workers encounter affect and are affected by more than one institution or system, there are frequent occasions on which interorganizational committees and meetings are relevant and appropriate as part of clinical social work practice. One example is work with delinquent youth, where the school system, the police department, and juvenile services administration might all be involved. If the family is in counseling in a community mental health center, that adds yet another component. Another example is a situation of ongoing domestic violence where, in addition to the police, there are professionals involved who represent a shelter for abused women and an alcohol treatment center, respectively. These are both the kinds of clinical cases that might be discussed in an administrative meeting.

Many social workers, of course, serve full-time in administrative capacities and participate in a wide variety of meetings on a daily basis. These vary from small staff meetings of a few individuals working on a given project to countywide or statewide or national committees or commissions made up of people from many organizations and agencies. Such groups are often formed to plan or implement a major program. For other social workers, participation in an administrative meeting consists primarily of staff and staff committee meetings, with occasional membership in a group with broader membership and issues.

It seems a fair observation that much less attention has been paid to the skills associated with membership, leadership, and influence in administrative groups than in those concerned with treatment (Ephross and Vassil, 1988; Falck, 1988). As a natural concomitant, for reasons poorly understood and little studied, both administrators and clinicians frequently leave their group work skills at the door when entering an agency or interorganizational meeting, because they identify the group work skills they learned only with client groups. In fact, all groups may be viewed as having a double set of purposes. The work of the group and the needs of individual members need to be addressed in administrative groups as well as in all others. At the same time, it may well be that membership in administrative groups demands a higher level of socialization to the demands of groups in general and of this type of group in particular. One reason this is true is that in groups formed for administrative purposes, the ability of the group to accomplish goals may be limited to the extent that the group's resources are diverted to serve individualized needs of particular group members (Bernstein, 1993).

This chapter will demonstrate the importance–and appropriate use– of traditional group work skills in administrative groups, and will also delineate some of the special considerations that pertain to such settings. We will discuss some of the issues that confront administrative groups, as well as principles that can be applied in those settings.

ISSUES

People

A group worker may or may not have any control over the composition of an administrative group. For example, if it is an interorganizational group, the members may very well be appointed by their individual organizations without regard for what the final composition of the group will look like. Groups can be very much affected, however, by the age, race, and sex, as well as other critical factors such as the roles and statuses within their organizations, of the members. Workers should understand the implications of homogeneity and heterogeneity of the group's membership. If the worker has control, or at least some input, regarding the composition of the group, it is important to pay attention to ensuring diversity of membership, avoiding tokenism on the one hand and overload on the other.

It is particularly important to make sure that there are members who represent groups that will be affected by the decisions made. While this may appear obvious, there are some subtle ways in which this factor is often ignored. Group workers would not form a group whose purpose is to develop a program to prevent teen pregnancy in the inner city without having representation of the population to be served. However, it is not uncommon to find task groups formed to explore mechanisms for dealing with problems such as juvenile delinquency, with discussion focusing on the role of a variety of systems, including law enforcement, without anyone having thought to include a police official. Then, when one recommendation of the group is for police to be trained to deal differently with youth they arrest, everyone gets angry because the police resent and are resistant to the training.

> PRINCIPLE I: The composition of administrative groups has an impact not only on the dynamics and work of the group, but also on the ability of the group to implement its decisions.

Power and Conflict

An obvious way in which administrative groups differ from other groups is that the members are peers, not clients, of the staff member. This does not mean, however, that all members of the group have equal power. In a client group, all the power resides with the worker and the sponsoring organization. In an administrative group, if members represent different organizations and are at fairly comparable levels within their respective organizations, the power may be evenly distributed. The implications of the distribution of power can be considerable with regard to how the assignment of responsibilities and conflict is handled, the ability of the group to make a decision, and the ability of the group to implement decisions. Members are peers, so the worker's ability to influence how conflicts are resolved is limited and depends on group history, links between representatives and sponsoring organizations, and other factors. Who has access to resources? What is at stake for the members, individually and collectively, if the group succeeds or fails at its goal? These questions combine with issues of personality and management style to affect outcomes of conflict over both process and products of administrative groups.

PRINCIPLE II: The distribution of power in an administrative group strongly influences the nature of conflict and how it is resolved, as well as how decisions are made and carried out.

Politics

All administrative groups are political in nature. Members and staff ignore this fact at their peril. On the simplest level, a group's goals and activities can have implications for the careers of its members. Beyond that, what a group does can have implications for the organizations or agencies represented, as well as for their constituencies or organizational entities at the broadest level. Consider the example of an interorganizational group planning a national conference, funded in part by a federal government grant, on strategies to address drug abuse and violence among youth. Any or all of the following might be discussed: whether to have as a speaker a convicted felon who discusses how he got involved with drugs and crime; whether it would be appropriate to have a cash bar as part of a dinner reception; the implications of inviting senators and representatives known to be good speakers, but clearly identified with particular bills that are pending in Congress on the issues involved; and how to determine who will select and who will invite those asked to serve as keynote speakers. If the political implications of decisions made by the group are not considered overtly, they will exert all the more influence covertly.

Groups are symbolic entities, and politics is a symbolic process. As Gummer (1987) has reminded us, the symbolic processes within a group always have interpersonal, organizational, and (often) macrosocial meanings as well. Sensitivity to these symbolic meanings is one of the marks of a skilled administrator in a group, as it is the mark of a skilled organizational representative. This sensitivity is a legitimate skill, often learned by trial and error over a long period of years. Too often, the question of symbolic meaning and political skill in groups has been treated as somehow illicit, or mysterious. It is neither, and deserves study in the light of day.

PRINCIPLE III: Every aspect of administrative groups has political implications.

Participation

The link between participation in decisions and identification with implementing them is one of the firmest products of small group research (Mulder, 1973). It is critical that members of an administrative group participate actively in the decision-making process. If only a few members attend meetings or share in the discussion of proposed actions, it is very difficult to gain the involvement of the nonparticipatory members in carrying out any activities decided upon. Successful implementation of decisions requires that members identify with and feel ownership of those decisions.

PRINCIPLE IV: People feel identification with and, hence, commitment to and responsibility for, decisions that they see themselves as having had a role in making.

Purpose

The accomplishment of the goals of a group is critical. If the group does not attain its goals, it ceases to exist. Satisfaction with group process, in this sense, takes a back seat to the productivity of an administrative group. Once decisions are made, a clear delineation of responsibility must be decided upon by group members in order to ensure that all aspects of follow-up are planned. Roles should be discussed, acknowledged, and agreed to. A major cause of failure of groups is agreement regarding a plan of action without any provision for having the action take place. To be successful, groups need to enlist the support of both the group's members and the organizations they represent.

PRINCIPLE V: Groups need to accomplish at least a portion of their goals.

CRITICAL GROUP WORK SKILLS

Given the issues and principles identified above, what skills can group workers bring to administrative groups that facilitate their success?

1. Provide input to ensure as broad a representation as possible among the members of the group, given the goals and issues involved.
2. When seemingly irrational behavior is exhibited on the part of a member, respond from the point of view of the group as a whole, so that the group's process can continue without being subverted. Do not forget your clinical understandings, nor the importance of the balances between containment and expression, strategic thinking and transparency.
3. Identify the members of the group who command respect and exhibit leadership, and work with them to ensure that the focus of the group stays on the goals.
4. When conflict arises, let the group deal with it. If it cannot or will not, influence the group by suggesting one or more nonthreatening explanations that allow the members involved to depersonalize the tension and either resolve the conflict or move on.
5. Be aware of both individual and organizational political agendas. Help keep the group focused on making decisions that accomplish the stated mission and goals without putting members or their organizations in the untenable position of having the group's decisions compromise the members' individual or organizational agendas.
6. Involve people. Use bridging and synthesizing techniques. Recognize contributions of members. Encourage the greatest level of participation possible on the part of members.
7. Remember and reflect in your behaviors in the group the mutual interdependence between goals and group process. Without at least some level of goal attainment, the process is generally experienced as meaningless. Without at least some level of satisfaction with group process, the accomplishments of a group will be transitory and the commitment of the group members to implementing decisions will be limited, at best. Workers should facilitate group accomplishment of goals by being supportive of productivity, by being technically facilitative, and by encouraging delineation of responsibilities that ensure that actions and activities will be implemented.

8. Take some responsibility for the emotional climate of the group. Use humor, perspective, and support to help maintain the morale of the group and help it achieve its goals.

The framework of practice principles and skills suggested here, like so much of group work and, indeed, all of social work skills, is both soundly based and in need of further empirical testing. The accomplishments of group work, which has always occupied a small minority position within social work, testify to the accumulated practice wisdom of its practitioners and to the ubiquity of small groups as social forms. The paucity of empirical evidence on the outcomes of group work in administration defines a research agenda for the present and the future.

REFERENCES

Bernstein, S. (1993). Personal communication to the authors, November 16.
Brown, L. N. (1991). *Groups for Growth and Change.* New York: Longman.
Ephross, P. H. (1981). Group work with work groups–A case of arrested development. *Social Work with Groups,* 4, 2.
Ephross, P. H. & Vassil, T. V. (1988). *Groups that Work: Structure and Process.* New York: Columbia University Press.
_____ . (1993). The rediscovery of real-world groups, in Wenocur, S., Ephross, P. H., Vassil, T. V., and Varghese, R. K. eds. *Group Work: Expanding Horizons.* New York: The Haworth Press, Inc.
Falck, H. (1988). *Social Work: The Membership Perspective.* New York: Springer Publishing Company.
Garvin, C. (1987). *Contemporary Group Work, 2nd ed.* Englewood Cliffs, NJ: Prentice-Hall.
Gummer, B. (1987). Groups as substance and symbol: Group processes and organizational politics. *Social Work with Groups,* 10, 2.
Mulder, M. (1973). Communication structure, decision structure and group performance, in Ofshe, R. J., ed. *Interpersonal Behavior in Small Groups.* Englewood Cliffs, NJ: Prentice Hall.
Toseland, R. W. & Ephross, P. H., eds. (1987). *Working Effectively with Administrative Groups.* New York: The Haworth Press, Inc.
Toseland, R. W. & Rivas, R. (1984). *An Introduction to Group Work Practice.* New York: Macmillan.

Chapter 5

The Dual-Purpose Group: Its Use and Misuse in Group Work Education

Cyrus S. Behroozi

It can be assumed that the success of group work practice, particularly in dealing with complex problems of our troubled society, is directly related to the effectiveness of group work education. An important part of group work education is experiential learning opportunities (Euster, 1979), which increasingly include dual-purpose groups (e.g., Oxley et al., 1979; Berger, 1992). Although the use of such groups in group work education is not yet pervasive, in many other human service professions, preparation of students for work with groups includes participation in a dual-purpose group. For example, in an exhaustive review of the literature (Dies, 1980), this type of group has been identified as one of four components in the training of group psychotherapists. A more recent study (Huhn et al., 1985) has found that 80 percent of counselor education programs surveyed used such a group.

In group work education, a dual-purpose group is composed of students enrolled in a group work course. The group experience serves two interrelated purposes, one *functional* and the other *instructional* (Behroozi, 1984). The functional purpose is to provide students with an experience of working as a group on a common problem, and the instructional purpose is to help them learn from the experience concepts and principles of group dynamics and group work practice. In terms of their functional purpose, dual-purpose group may deal with task problems (e.g., planning a class presentation) or with members' personal problems. The latter dual-purpose groups is the primary focus of this chapter.

In the past decade, the author regularly included dual-purpose groups in his graduate group work course. The discussion that follows is primarily based on his extensive evaluations of the groups, his struggle with the issues that emerged from the evaluations, and his search for ways of dealing with the issues.

USE OF THE DUAL-PURPOSE GROUP

As an experiential learning opportunity, the dual-purpose groups formed by the author were intended to engage the course students in the phenomena studied (Kendall et al., 1986) and to establish an environment for their active participation (Waldie, 1982). The conceptual framework for the group experience was the learning cycle model developed by Kolb and Fry (1975). As shown by Figure 5.1, this cycle consists of four stages. In the first stage, the learner is involved in a concrete, here-and-now experience. In the second

FIGURE 5.1

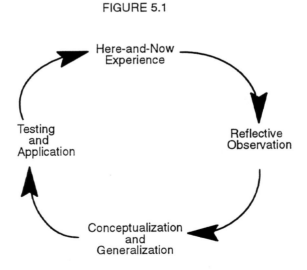

stage, through reflective observation, relevant phenomena are selected from the experience. In the third stage, such phenomena are analyzed, conceptualized, and generalized in relation to theoretical knowledge. Finally, the concepts and principles formulated in the third stage are tested and applied in new situations, which may constitute the beginning of a new cycle. Thus, the learning cycle can continuously recur since learned concepts and principles may be modified in new experiences.

The dual-purpose groups in the course served as the first stage (concrete, here-and-now experience) in the cycle. For the second stage (reflective observation), the students engaged in process analysis and journal writing after each session of the group. Activities for the third stage (conceptualization and generalization of observations) included class discussions and readings. For the fourth stage (testing and application), the students prepared a term paper synthesizing their learning and applied it to practice with a group anticipated for their next semester's field practicum.

The functional purpose of the groups was to help the student-members deal with selected problems experienced in their professional education. The instructional purpose of the groups was to facilitate the students' achievement of several objectives related to the group work course: (1) to test theoretical concepts about group process, (2) to test principles of group work practice, (3) to increase self-awareness for group work practice, (4) to develop empathy for the client-member role, (5) to develop appreciation for the worker role, and (6) to develop skills for group work practice.

Typically, following the introductory session of the course, the students discussed the process of group formation. At the same time, they were asked to identify, in writing, issues that they wanted to address in their group and concerns that they had about participation in the group. Based on the students' interests, sections of the group were formed to meet for eight weekly sessions of about one hour and 15 minutes during the class time. Every group session was followed by a processing period, after which all students assembled in the class to discuss theoretical concepts and principles.

During the first few years, the course instructor served as the worker for the dual-purpose groups. However, because of a host of logistical and other problems, the leadership of the groups was eventually left to the students.

Systematic evaluations of the dual-purpose groups (Behroozi, 1984, 1987, 1988, 1989) consistently evidenced their success in terms of the students' achievement of the instructional objectives. The only exception was adequate development of skills for practice with groups.

POTENTIAL MISUSE OF THE DUAL-PURPOSE GROUP

The early evaluations of the dual-purpose groups primarily focused on the instructional objectives and did not consider "unanticipated effects" (West and Kirkland, 1986) of the group experience. Gradually, attention was drawn to the following unanticipated effects as the bases for the potential misuse of the dual-purpose group.

1. *Substitution for Field Practicum.* The author's dual-purpose groups were offered in a semester that did not include a field practicum experience. Primarily because of this, one of the instructional objectives of the groups was to help the students develop practice skills. However, as already noted, the students' achievement of this objective was inadequate. In fact, as evidenced by one of the evaluations of the group experience (Behroozi, 1989), the students' professional self-esteem, and thus their readiness to embark on practice with groups, actually diminished as a result of the experience. Apparently, the reason was that while the students had become aware of the requirements for effective group work practice, they did not have an opportunity for testing and validating their ability to meet the requirements. In other words, they had learned *about* the group worker role without being able *to act in* the role. The process of acting in the role can be completed only by an encounter with a "real" group in field practicum or in other practice situations. This conclusion is consistent with that reached by Mary Huntington (1957) in her classic study of the development of the professional self-image of a group of medical students: ". . . students who felt they handled the problems

of their assigned families without difficulty showed a greater tendency to develop this professional self-image . . . " (p. 187).

In some social work education programs, the difficulty of developing appropriate group work field practicum opportunities has led to the substitution of the dual-purpose group for field practicum. This substitution is implicitly justified by the cynical "better-than-nothing" rationale. However, as also concluded by Kacen and Soffer (1990), while the dual-purpose group can be a viable experience for learning practice concepts and principles, it cannot serve as a substitution for field practicum, which is indispensable for developing practice skills.

2. *Education vs. Therapy.* In spite of the author's efforts to clarify the functional purpose of the dual-purpose groups, a recurring question–and concern–on the part of the students was whether that purpose was therapy or education. In considering such a question, Zinberg and Shapiro (1963) have asserted that "therapy at its best is not necessarily different from education at its best," especially if the latter is to bring forth or mature capabilities in individuals. This position is arguable, because a lack of distinction between therapy and education as the central focus of the dual-purpose group can be potentially harmful to the group members. For example, this potential can exist even when the group experience includes such a common objective as development of students' self-awareness. Achieving this objective may involve unpacking, if not breaking down, some of the students' psychological defenses. What are the consequences of this unpacking of students' defenses? If the consequences require therapeutic counseling, how should it be provided? Generally, should any component of a group work course be designed as a therapeutic experience? Is this indicated in the course syllabus, which constitutes the contract between the instructor and students?

3. *Involuntary Participation.* Although the importance of voluntary participation in groups has been stressed from the ethical (Bernstein, 1976), motivational (Behroozi, 1992), and therapeutic (Yalom, 1975) standpoints, participation in the author's

dual-purpose groups, as in other such experiences in group work education, was mandatory. This was justified by an assumption that, because of the students' "free choice" of social work education, they enroll in social work courses and participate in course activities voluntarily (Falck, 1992). However, the author's assessments of the perception of the student-members of the dual-purpose groups pointed out that many of them entered the groups involuntarily, that is, for reasons not of their own choosing. Such a perception is a serious problem in any area of professional education, considering that students, as adult learners, need opportunities for active, self-directed learning (Boud, 1988). The perception is particularly serious in group work education because of its emphasis on democratic principles and group members' self-determination. As Valli (1990) has stated, if students' educational experience does not represent principles taught, they can hardly be expected to develop adequate commitment to the implementation of the principles in their professional practice. More specifically, Kacen and Soffer (1990) have argued that student members' involuntary participation in class groups severely impairs the function of class modeling for group work practice.

4. *Peer-Leader's Competence.* This issue is primarily relevant to the peer-led group, which is the most prevalent model of dual-purpose groups in group work education (e.g., Berger, 1992; Oxley et al., 1979). The author's experience suggests that inherent in peer leadership of the dual-purpose group is the serious problem that a student-leader typically does not possess the necessary skills to help the group members deal with all content generated in the group experience. A significant example of such content is personal issues inappropriately disclosed by the group members who do not understand the boundary of the group or who are unable to limit their participation to the boundary.

5. *Dual-Role Relationships.* Another major issue constituting a basis for the potential misuse of the dual-purpose group is dual-role relationships. In instructor-led dual-purpose groups, the dual-role relationship between the instructor-worker and student-members can be a fertile ground for exploitation and

manipulation by the instructor who holds dual power over students and by students who can frustrate the instructor in dual ways (Thompson, 1990). In student-led dual-purpose groups, such a relationship may lead to a conflict between the group leader role and the leader's personal relationships with some of the group members (Oxley et al., 1979).

IMPLICATIONS AND RECOMMENDATIONS

There is strong evidence supporting the use of the dual-purpose group in group work education. Equally evident is the potential for its misuse. Unfortunately, the bases for the potential misuse of the group cannot be completely eliminated. Thus, the use of the dual-purpose group is justified only if its benefit clearly outweighs its risk for student-members (Hunt, 1990). This principle is the core of the ethical standards formulated by the Association for Specialists in Group Work (1989) for the use of the dual-purpose group in counseling education. Ultimately, such standards should also be developed for group work education. Meanwhile, to minimize the risk of the dual-purpose group, the following strategies are recommended for dealing with the bases for its potential misuse.

1. *Field Practicum.* At its best, the dual-purpose group is a vicarious experience. As such, it can serve as a link between conceptual learning in the classroom and practice experience in the field practicum. Thus, ideally, the dual-purpose group should be concurrent with field practicum. If this is not possible, the group experience should precede the field practicum. In either case, special efforts should be made to help students use the group experience to transfer their conceptual learning to the field practicum.

2. *Education vs. Therapy.* Both purposes of the dual-purpose group must be clearly linked to the course objectives. Thus, students' disclosure of personal issues in the group should be allowed only to the extent that these issues are related to their educational development. This characterization of the group content is similar to what Goldberg and Hartman (1984) have called "personal-professional" issues. These issues emerge

from the group members' own professional education experience as complicated by their contemporary personal circumstances. Examples of these issues include conflicts between the members' student role and their other roles, such as employee, spouse, and parent. Furthermore, the group's treatment of these issues must be limited to supportive problem-solving.

3. *Involuntary Participation.* As prescribed by Yalom (1975), participation in the dual-purpose group should be voluntary. Therefore, the group must be clearly described in the course syllabus distributed among prospective students before their enrollment in the course. The dual-purpose group should be discussed with prospective students, particularly focusing on its purpose, expectations, and rationale (Pierce and Baldwin, 1990). Furthermore, meaningful alternatives to the dual-purpose group should be provided for students who need to take the course but are unwilling to participate in the group.

4. *Peer Leader's Competence.* Forester-Miller and Duncan (1990) have recommended that peer leadership of the dual-purpose group be allowed only if the professional person responsible for the group (e.g., the course instructor) can be present in the group sessions. However, it is more practical for the instructor to monitor the group sessions regularly in order to provide consultation for the peer-leader and, if necessary, to intervene immediately. Examples of strategies for monitoring the group sessions include the instructor's participation in the processing of the group sessions and review of student-members' journals. In any case, the instructor should try to prevent harmful disclosures in the group sessions by making sure that, from the beginning, members of the group are clear about its purpose and boundary, and about examples of appropriate and inappropriate content for discussion in the group.

5. *Dual-Role Relationships.* Kitchener (1988) has identified certain obligations for any professional person in dual-role relationships. Accordingly, if the course instructor leads the dual-purpose group, the instructor is required to be aware of the possible conflict between the dual roles, to clarify for student-members the different expectations associated with each role, and to minimize the conflict by developing procedures for

safeguarding students' interests. An example of such a procedure is that students' participation in the group is not graded. If the dual-purpose group is led by student-peers, to the appropriate extent, the instructor should explain these obligations to the group and should monitor their implementation.

REFERENCES

Association for Specialists in Group Work (1989). *Ethical Guidelines for Group Counselors.* Alexandria, VA: Author.

Behroozi, C. (1984). A model for systematic teaching of group work. Paper presented at the Annual Symposium for the Advancement of Social Work with Groups, Chicago.

_____ . (1987). A socialization group in education for group work. Paper presented at the CSWE Annual Program Meeting, St. Louis.

_____ . (1988). Outcomes of student support groups in relation to three leadership patterns. Paper presented at the Annual Symposium for the Advancement of Social Work with Groups, Baltimore.

_____ . (1989). Effects of group experience on the professional self-esteem of group work students. In *Proceedings of the 11th Symposium on Social Work with Groups,* Montreal.

_____ . (1992). Groupwork with involuntary clients: Remotivating strategies. *Groupwork, 5,* 31-41.

Berger, B. (1992). Doing, watching and documenting: The use of lab groups and task group observation in teaching group work theory and skills. Paper presented at the Annual Symposium for the Advancement of Social Work with Groups, Atlanta.

Bernstein, S. (1976). Values and group work. In S. Bernstein (Ed.), *Further Explorations in Group Work.* Boston: Charles River.

Boud, D. (1988). *Developing Student Autonomy in Learning.* London: Kogan Page.

Dies, R. (1980). Current practice in the training of group psychotherapists. *International Journal of Group Psychotherapy, 30,* 160-185.

Euster, G. (1979). Trends in education for social work practice with groups. *Journal of Education for Social Work, 15,* 94-99.

Falck, H. (1992). Teaching group work (Letter). *Journal of Teaching in Social Work, 6,* 189-191.

Forester-Miller, H. & Duncan, J. (1990). The ethics of dual relationships in the training of group counselors. *Journal for Specialists in Group Work, 15,* 88-93.

Goldberg, T. & Hartman, C. (1984). The lab experience: The class as a context for learning about groups. *Social Work with Groups, 7,* 67-84.

Huhn, R., Zimpfer, D., Waltman, D., & Williamson, S. (1985). A survey of programs of professional preparation for group counseling. *The Journal for Specialists in Group Work, 10,* 124-133.

Hunt, J. (1990). *Ethical Issues in Experiential Education.* Boulder, CO: The Association for Experiential Education.

Huntington, M. (1957). The development of a professional self-image. In R. Merton, G. Reader, & P. Kendall (Eds.), *The Student Physician.* Cambridge: Harvard University Press.

Kacen, L. & Soffer, S. (1990). Coping with contradictory messages in training group workers. *Journal of Teaching in Social Work, 4,* 53-66.

Kendall, J., Duley, J., Little, T., Purmaul, J., & Rubin, S. (1986). *Strengthening Experiential Education.* Raleigh, NC: National Society for Internship and Experiential Education.

Kitchener, K. (1988). Dual role relationships: What makes them so problematic? *Journal of Counseling and Development, 67,* 217-221.

Kolb, D. & Fry, D. (1975). *Toward an Applied Theory of Experiential Learning.* In C. Cooper (Ed.), *Theories of Group Process.* New York: John Wiley.

Oxley, G., Wilson, S., Anderson, J., & Wong, S. (1979). Peer-led groups in graduate education. *Social Work with Groups, 2,* 67-76.

Pierce, K. & Baldwin, C. (1990). Participation versus privacy in the training of group counselors. *The Journal for Specialists in Group Work, 15,* 149-158.

Thompson, A. (1990). *Guide to Ethical Practice in Psychotherapy.* New York: John Wiley and Son.

Waldie, K. (1982). Experiential learning groups: An application model. *Small Group Behavior, 13,* 75-90.

West, A. & Kirkland, M. (1986). Effectiveness of growth groups in education. *Journal for Specialists in Group Work, 11,* 16-24.

Valli, L. (1992). Beginning teacher problems: Areas for teacher education improvement. *Action in Teacher Education, 14,* 18-25.

Yalom, I. (1975). *The Theory and Practice of Group Psychotherapy* (2nd Ed.). New York: Basic Books

Zinberg, N. & Shapiro, D. (1963). A group approach in contexts of therapy and education. *Mental Hygiene, 47,* 108-116.

Chapter 6

Central Characteristics
of Social Work with Groups–
A Sociocultural Analysis

Hans S. Falck

INTRODUCTION

We are in the middle of a long historical process that has robbed
the professions of what once upon a time seemed to be tacit and
unquestioned confidence in our judgement. All professions are involved here; no longer does the assumption reign that the professional person, on account of both calling and education, knows, and
knows better than the lay public, what ails the latter, and how to
cure it. Medicine is only the most prominent among such groups,
but few are omitted from the scrutiny of ever more knowledgeable
clients. People want to know what we do, why we do it, how well
trained we are to perform it, and how we differ from others claiming
the same or related skill and authority and the ability to collect
money for our efforts.

Thus, professional work has been robbed of its mystique, with
the sun shining glaringly on our efforts and on their results. Insofar
as social work and social work with groups are concerned, the main
issue is not what makes us unique among competing professions.
The real question has to do with centrality, that is, what does our
training and experience qualify us to offer the public, and what are
the essential characteristics of that which make it social work, and
in our case, social work with groups. We are called upon to be clear
and precise rather than absolutely right. Yet, clarity and precision

are in very short supply and the effort before us is one attempt to furnish some of that rare commodity.

The argument to be presented here is made with respect for and in consonance with the overall title of this volume, *Group Work Practice in a Troubled Society: Problems and Opportunities*. It is a framework one does not take lightly, for the troubled society is our society. That troubled state affects each and every human being, and in particular, the clients we work with. We can say, therefore, that social workers and clients are members of that same troubled world, a world largely of our own making.

Social work with groups is not new to the troubled society. The aim from the very outset was and ought to remain the betterment of our common social life and the building of the competence of each and every client member who comes to our attention. The literature on the subject is very specific. The aims and goals of early social work, including social work with groups, was to better peoples *social* conditions together with other people suffering similar disadvantages. In this spirit, the task before us is to cast our eyes on the present condition of our methodology, its values, its underlying assumptions, and its practitioners. It is *not* to introduce a practice police that determines, at the pain of retribution, what social workers should or should not do. What it does propose is to introduce a newly reasoned, principled view of what kinds of group work practice appear to be consistent with social work's mission.

The most recent stage in the ongoing debate about the nature of group work and its purposes is to be credited to the painstaking work by Ted Goldberg (1991, 1992) of Wayne State University. In two papers Professor Goldberg has summarized and discussed in great detail the national discussion about the topics already mentioned. Both papers evoked profound discussion in the meetings where they were given and the 1992 presentation offered the further advantage of a section on "Definitions and Distinctions" that reflected the thoughts of many senior writers and scholars in the field. But rather than redo Goldberg's work, we shall pose his questions in a somewhat different way, and try to understand what it is that influences our decision making about our most defining concepts.

In thinking about social work with groups one is assisted by similar considerations for the profession of social work as a whole.

We are not nearly as distant from our parent profession as it might seem at first glance, given social work's preoccupation with clinical, ruggedly individualistic assumptions, and its ever more marginal interest–primarily in the case of direct practice personnel–in social process, social action, and community change. Similarly, what disturbs many in the profession about these tendencies is hardly absent in group work discussions, though it should be acknowledged that the programming of the Association for the Advancement of Social Work with Groups consistently offers papers on the social action aspects of social group work, and a recent special issue of *Social Work with Groups* (Vinik and Levin, 1991) appeared under the title of "Social Action in Group Work."

A SOCIOCULTURAL ANALYSIS

The difficulties and the shortcomings in social work practice and education, including social work with groups, are no mere accident of history. Nor are they traceable to the suggestion that somehow social workers are less capable than other professionals when it comes to defining their roles. Instead, the problems are to be found deeply embedded in American and Western culture, in the sociology of the professions in general, in the class structure of social work, and in the desires, hopes, and expectations of social workers choosing the profession in the first place.

The literature on the early days of social work in general and including social group work says that to reach legitimation and currently valid answers for what troubles our clients is to make the method deal with individuals and with groups at the same time, and to use the group as a mechanism for personal growth. The secondary theme is that if individuals do well, so will groups, since, so the assumptions runs, groups consist of individuals. The term for this, taken from modern philosophy, is *methodological individualism,* a bitterly controversial topic based on the claim that all social life reduces to the individual (Lukes, 1973).

But it is also true that the clinical literature in social work reaches back to the early American Freudians. Its tone from the very beginning was and remains to this day one shared with those others who diagnose and treat emotional and psychiatric illness. The entire history of medical and medically influenced practice in the Western world focuses on the biological core of the individual, one by one. Although there exists a small and at the same time powerful literature (and first-rate theoretical work) in psychosomatic medicine, it does not take into consideration social aspects of living. Holism, the doctrine of the interrelatedness of human life, remains–as does group work–on the cultural defensive in the face of various doctrines of individualism (James, 1984). In general, the insistence on individualism as primary concern and collectivism as secondary theme has left both thought and social work practice unintegrated, especially so since the one supersedes the other as the basic alternative.

As clinically focused social work became ever more dominant–nearly always conceived of as with or in behalf of individuals even when spoken of in group terms–social group work lost a great deal of its preferential relevance. Group therapy and family therapy to this day most often replace social group work in social work education. Yet, what has been lost is less the significance of the methodology of social group work than the reasons and the logic of social work with groups in a philosophical sense. In terms of the latter, the essential message earlier in our history was that informal learning under guided enablement by social group workers could offer each person the help needed to increase their social competences while at the same time learning to use groups to influence their common lives. This was Grace Coyle's message in light of the well-known influence of John Dewey upon her thought.

What is being described here anticipated to some extent membership theory in social work, although both Dewey and Coyle were individualists. In membership theory, however, the central construct is the human member, whereas in the tradition of social work with groups, as well as clinical social work and the therapies, the fundamental construct is the life of the individual. Within this same set of assumptions the group is a collectivity, while within membership theory the group equals its members. I know of no method outside of social work that claims this latter territory, the nature of human membership, as its central concern.

In sum, social work conceptualization based on scientific fact, with its overriding concern with individuals and collectivities of individuals, has come to a halt and thereby offers little current basis for the enormous amounts of social change necessary in American society. The individualistic focus of so-called treatment strategies at the center of social work with groups or any other social work method documents this trend.

To answer questions about the reasons for the state of affairs described it would seem necessary to consider the following:

1. Social work's preoccupation with radical individualism consistent with the same preference in American life in general; and on a conceptual level with methodological individualism.
2. That the primary message university-centered professional education proclaims is the desirability of the improvement of each individual conceptualized as the self even to the point of graduating clearly unsuitable workers while ignoring the harm this potentially does to clients. Rationales range from being personally troubled to being entitled to another chance. The middle-class aspirations of students seeking a profession often take precedence over the rights of clients to superior quality services.
3. That the distortion of the meaning of advanced education as a right stresses entitlements of students without attention or lacking attention to the social good. The resistance to supervision and the demand that all work be graded "A" are only some examples.
4. Social work theories and research are characterized by the same methodological individualism already touched upon, the latter a doctrine in the philosophy of science which holds that all human action including that in groups and in society can be reduced to individual behavior.
5. The bypassing and ignoring of research findings stressing interactionism rather than individualistic if not simplistic assumptions about causation.
6. The denigration of educative experience in small groups, substituting the assumption that human disability is to be understood as either individual victimization or individual sickness requiring therapy.
7. The dominance of the role of the professional, not as enabler, but as expert in curing what besets individuals. It is clearly the role of the therapist as expert in the causes and cures of human suffering.

68

Some reflection on this list of social work proclivities results in the serious conclusion that American social work is syntonic with serious weaknesses in American culture in general, making social work ever more acceptable to most of the population at the cost of dropping its social responsibilities. Its concern with the expertise of the professional, with ideological individualism, with methodological individualism in research and theory building, and with the advancement of the professional into academically validated middle-class status are all part and parcel of dominant American thought. In fact, social work has arrived within the framework of American assumptions about the role of the professional person in general.

One major attempt to come to terms with the individualistic preoccupations in the profession was ecological social work, heavily promoted in the field and embraced by NASW and many others of the person-in-situation formulation. Those aspects of systems or ecological approaches dominated as much in group work practice as in clinical practice–most often referred to in systems terms–and still do so. While the specific language differs somewhat depending on the method one discusses, whatever the language or framework, it in no way diminishes the rank individualism of social work, including social work with groups (Falck, 1991). It adds the environment to the individual and sometimes the group, and thereby fails to analyze the dysfunctionality of both. The author's work on membership theory addresses the issues involved in detail (Falck, 1988, 1989).

Tied to these currents has been the improvement of the social status of social work practitioners. One may currently enter the profession with full assurance that the work is as respectable as most other professions. Most people understand quite readily what is meant by diagnosing and treating–there are sufficient reminders from their medical experience as patients. In addition, keeping things confidential between one therapist and one patient reassures the client that he/she is the only one who has the ear of the social worker in the guise of the doctor model. Therapists and patients benefit, as Parsons said long ago, from a certain mystique implicit in the former's expertise (Parsons, 1951).

To the degree that social work with groups insists on the perpetuation of the model of informal education–in Europe typically named social pedagogy–that gave rise to it, and to the extent that through its methodology it protests and rejects the rugged individualism expressed in mindless competition, be it in the lives of clients or among social work clinicians competing for paying patients, it becomes suspect and is rejected by social workers–often dominant in national councils and in powerful professional associations–and is substituted for by more comforting labels. The near demise of conscious social change through social work groups is no dictate of history, but has resulted from the fact that social workers, including social group workers, have increasingly embraced the dominant American preoccupation with the individual self.

SOCIAL WORK WITH GROUPS: SUGGESTED CRITERIA

The essence of social work with groups, be it through social group work or in task-oriented groups, should be consistent with a clear view of the social work profession. In our view all of the following standards must be met in order for the work of the social worker to be social work and to be social work with groups.

1. The work is social work and thereby social work with groups when clients teach each other (i.e., learn from each other) how to meet their human needs through democratic group process under social work auspices.
2. The work is social work when the aim of social group work activity is to *assist* clients to teach each other.
3. It is social work and social work with groups when social workers and social agencies commit each other to the intention of helping each and all members of the group to perform in consonance with *their own and others needs at the same time* (Falck, 1984, 1988, 1989), including conflict resolution work and the recognized need for individuation (not individualization) within the membership group.
4. It is social work with groups when social workers and agencies commit themselves to help members of a group learn from each other as well as from and through the worker how to bring about change *outside* their group.
5. The work is social work when clients are constantly helped to become conscious of the ethically and scientifically docu-

mented fact that the behaviors of all persons have significant consequences for others, both in and outside the group.

We stress the idea of commitment by social workers and agencies, not only to point up what it takes to do social work with groups but also to name some indicators which suggest observability and therefore accountability for the work done.

WHAT IS NOT *SOCIAL WORK WITH GROUPS*

The work is *not* social work when:

1. The purpose is change in the individual self without constant reference to and involvement of other members (often referred to as casework with an audience) or regard for them; and
2. The group is used essentially as the occasion for personal/individual gain; and
3. The social worker is referred to as the leader of the group and behaves accordingly, making the clients followers of the leader by definition; and
4. The standard method of understanding member behavior and intervention is couched in terms of psychopathology and treatment; and
5. Social change and social action are by-products, incidental to the main content of the group membership experience.

All of these are the characteristics of what is not social work with groups as viewed and understood by the author of this chapter.

The applications of what we have identified as criteria for social work practice, including social work practice with groups, are put forth as being able to help us answer what belongs in social work and what does not. The criteria for inclusion in or exclusion from social work are consistent with both scientific and ethical implications of membership theory (Falck, 1989). Social work with groups rejects the split between the individual and the group, as I view it. It supports individuation of members *within the group*. It affirms thereby man's biosocial nature as irreducible–a sharp turn away from traditional individualism.

It is incumbent upon social workers, and group workers specifically, to recognize that what began as individuation within groups has ended with individualization as the alternative to membership behavior, to the major exclusion of a civic spirit, and to the unabated rejection of social values other than the quick fix and money oriented, cut throat competition in and outside the professions. People in this country cry out for leadership which holds to the very ideals that social group workers in the long tradition of the method have espoused, and the weakening of which has had much to do with the near demise of the social pedagogic and social action contributions social workers have made.

There is a price, then, that is paid when the tacit message is that what ails our clients (and us) is to be explained in terms of individualism, the conversion of every human need into an absolute individual right, and in a civic violence that ignores what we owe each other as members of the human community. All this has become somewhat attenuated thanks to the civil rights movement and those efforts aiming at a more just life for women. What has not been addressed is the violence of men in their relationship among themselves, especially in business and industry, nor the incipient violence in the authority-dictated hierarchies in our own profession and others in which men play dominant roles to this day.

We suggest that a huge step toward the humanization of small group life in family, in business, in the professions, and elsewhere can be made if the normative structure of American society would permit sensitivity, the expression of positive feelings, and a less competitive life-style by and among men. It is a task perfectly fitted for social work with groups, in which membership, connectedness, affection, and the expression of the real self are valued, supported, and praised. It might indeed lead to a society in which taxpayers and those who voluntarily provide for others in need see their ability to give of themselves as a strength, instead of as a loss endured voluntarily or through force. It is a task clearly worthy of the social work profession and of social group workers in particular.

CONCLUDING QUESTIONS

Should group psychotherapy be considered social work? Were there a definition of group psychotherapy available, clear and consistent, the question could be answered directly. There is no such definition and, in fact, there exists a range of therapy types, running from the openly individualistic to the group-as-a-whole type of work, all claiming success. What we have attempted to supply in this chapter are ways and criteria which would help answer the question, and their application would surely do so. Yet, the overriding concern is not with the relatively minor question about the nature of group psychotherapy; rather, it is with the major question about the nature and the future of professional social work with groups. That, in the face of our troubled society, is worthy of our best effort.

REFERENCES

Falck, H. S. (1984). The membership model of social work. *Social Work, 29*:2.

_____ (1988). *Social Work: The Membership Perspective,* New York: Springer Publishing Company.

_____ (1989). The management of membership: Social group work contributions. *Social Work with Groups, 12*:3.

_____ (1991). The concepts *individual* and *group* in social group work theory: a fifty-year review. Paper presented at the 13th Annual Meeting of the Association for the Advancement of Social Work with Groups, Akron, OH. Unpublished–available from the author.

Goldberg, T. (1991). Group work and group treatment: A preliminary analysis. Paper presented at the 13th Annual Meeting of the Association for the Advancement of Social Work with Groups, Akron, OH.

_____ (1992). Beliefs and attitudes about the group therapies by group workers. Paper presented at the 14th Annual Meeting of the Association for the Advancement of Social Work with Groups, Atlanta, GA.

James, S. (1984). *The Content of Social Explanation,* Cambridge: Cambridge University Press.

Lukes, S. (1973). *Individualism,* Oxford: Basil Blackwell.

Parsons, T. (1951). *The Social System,* Glencoe, IL: The Free Press, pp. 450-451.

Vinik, A. and M. Levin, Guest Editors. (1991). Social action in group work, *Social Work with Groups, 14*:3/4.

Chapter 7

Using Group Work Skills to Promote Cultural Sensitivity Among Social Work Students

Elaine P. Congress
Maxine Lynn

INTRODUCTION

Teaching culturally sensitive practice and increasing self-awareness in this area are facilitated by an interactive group work approach. Addressing the role of the social work educator, both as a model and as a group leader, this chapter will focus on the use of group work skills to involve, educate, and empower diverse students within the classroom.

Social work educators have been concerned about effective teaching of culturally and racially diverse students (Gitterman, 1991; Manoleas and Carillo, 1991). They have been warned of the dangers of stereotyping (McGoldrick, Pearce, and Giordano, 1982), as well as of promoting ethnocentrism (Chau, 1990). Specific issues in working with African-American students (Gitterman, 1991) and Latino students (Manoleas and Carillo, 1991) have been addressed.

The social work profession has actively tried to recruit ethnically diverse students (Oliver and Brown, 1988). Nineteen percent of the current MSW school enrollment is described as belonging to an ethnic minority (Council on Social Work Education, 1990). In one east coast urban university, however, the enrollment of persons of color is closer to 30 percent.

Numerous opportunities to teach directly about cultural diversity arise from the classroom process. Yet teaching often becomes a mine field for social work educators who try to model cultural sensitivity.

LITERATURE REVIEW:
GROUPS AND CULTURAL DIVERSITY

Social group work has a long history of use with culturally diverse people. Groups were formed in settlement houses to help immigrants adjust to life in America (Brown, 1991). Originally, the purpose of groups with culturally diverse members seemed to be to promote assimilation. Currently, social workers have been concerned about a white-dominated ethnocentric approach (Lum, 1992). Respect for ethnic differences has recently led social group work to focus more on issues of mutual aid and self help (Gitterman and Shulman, 1986), promotion of ethnic identity and biculturalism (Chau, 1991), and empowerment (Solomon, 1976; Gutierrez and Ortega, 1991; Brown, 1991). The importance of augmenting client strengths in social group work practice with culturally diverse members has been identified (Brown, 1991; Lewis and Ford, 1991; Chau, 1991). While the power of groups in promoting ethnic-racial sensitivity (Glassman, 1991) and resolving interethnic conflict (Norman, 1991) has been noted, groups of mixed racial composition can be problematic to form and conduct (Davis and Proctor, 1989). In the social work literature there are limited examples of groups successfully brought together to promote interethnic harmony (Adams and Schlesinger, 1988; Latting, 1990).

The use of group work skills has been identified as significant in classroom teaching (Schwartz, 1964; Shulman, 1987). Not only in field work (Kadushin, 1992), but also in the classroom, the teacher as group leader emerges as an important role model. Students may be more influenced by what is "caught" than what is "taught" (Lewis, 1987). The importance of teacher style and use of professional self has been cited as crucial to student learning (Lewis, 1991). This is seen to be particularly significant in teaching culturally diverse students (Congress, 1992).

The group work skills discussed by Schwartz (1976), Brown (1991), and Shulman (1992) can be applied to the social work educator role within the classroom. The educator's tasks are to:

1. Explain the purpose of the class and reach for the common needs of students;
2. Negotiate a contract that clarifies the roles and responsibilities of teacher and students;
3. Develop a supportive culture in which students feel safe to participate;
4. Acknowledge and work through the impact of the authority of the teacher, as well as of student class leaders';
5. Tune in and work with the individual students in the class, as well as with the class as a whole;
6. Recognize and negotiate conflict; and
7. Build relationships and coalitions.

PURPOSE OF CLASS

During the beginning phase of group work, leaders should "explain and negotiate group purposes" (Brown, 1991) and answer "the clients' first question (which is) 'What are we here for?'" (Shulman, 1991). In social work education we perhaps erroneously make the assumption that everyone knows why he or she is in a particular class. It is not sufficient to expect that students will carefully read the class purpose that is usually delineated in printed material distributed to students. If oral communication is the primary method of student learning, then this should begin in the first class. This is particularly significant for culturally diverse students. Students in social work classes often have had very different educational experiences. Previous experience may have been in didactic classes in which the teacher lectured. For all students, social work education has more of an applied practice component than many other areas of study.

Group members always bring to a new group experience "old fears from early experiences" (Shulman, 1992, p. 316). This may be particularly true for culturally diverse students who often have had previously negative experiences within a white-dominated educational system (Pinderhughes, 1989). A clear statement of class purpose builds on common ground and helps everyone to begin at the same point. It is important for the instructor to scan the room, notice the seating patterns, and reach for each member's expectations. Often persons of color are huddled on the sides or in the back of the room.

Reaching for common needs is an essential part of group process and particularly important in promoting mutual respect among diverse students. To begin this process, faculty must tune into and examine their own beliefs about students. Do they have certain prejudices that students from particular ethnic groups may have more difficulty with the class material? Such beliefs are readily conveyed to culturally diverse students. Often the instructor's negative perception becomes a self-fulfilling prophecy.

It is expected that faculty will have their own prejudices and biases. In fact, to deny these beliefs is often dangerous, and promotes an "us and them" dichotomy. The instructor's openness that she/he too is a product of a certain background models for students the importance of self-awareness.

CONTRACTING–ROLES AND RESPONSIBILITIES

Contracting is an essential task in all social work practice and it is important that the social work educator model this behavior within the classroom. During this negotiating period in which both client and worker are involved, reaching for client feedback must occur (Shulman, 1992).

Contracting within the classroom involves defining the expected roles and responsibilities of both teacher and students. Important in all classroom teaching, this becomes particularly significant with a culturally diverse student group. American graduate education, especially in social work, usually involves an interactional approach which may be unfamiliar to many students. Some students may have anxiety about speaking up in class, especially if it is to question the authority of the teacher. Expected roles about class participation should be explicitly stated and negotiated from the very beginning in order to facilitate future classroom work and final evaluation of students' work.

Culturally diverse students often assume multiple roles as students, employees, spouses, family caretakers, and parents (Egan and Bombyk, 1991; Manoleas and Carillo, 1991). Therefore, responsibilities in terms of attendance and class assignments need a high degree of clarity. The nature of assignments should be discussed and the social work educator must be sure that all students understand expectations. Some students may be more familiar with academic writing skills than others, and the teacher must work to ensure that all students understand what is expected of them.

The teacher must reach for feedback about the contract negotiated with the class. Often, culturally diverse students may be reluctant to share their concerns about assignments, especially if the authority of the teacher might seem to be questioned. The teacher must encourage each student to ask questions about assignments. Sometimes misunderstandings arise, especially if English is the student's second language, as the following incident illustrates:

> In a practice class a bilingual student turned in a paper which contained a process recording of her work with a family in her field placement. The teacher had wanted the paper to be primarily theoretical, but had indicated that parts of the process could be used to illustrate the application of different family models to actual practice. The faculty member had failed to make clear to the class that the primary focus was theoretical and the student, fearful of expressing herself in front of the class, did not ask for clarification.

Contracting should include a statement that classroom incidents, whether subtle or overt, that reflect cultural and racial bias or concerns will be examined. Often these issues are quickly covered over by both the classroom process and the instructor. One reason may be social workers' value system, which stresses understanding and respect for all.

SUPPORTIVE CULTURE

The development of a supportive culture is essential in group work practice (Yalom, 1988). This also facilitates classroom learning in allowing students to feel free to participate. The social work educator must strive to promote respect and empower all class members, not only those who are the most verbal. All students should be encouraged to participate and share their experiences.

Students observe how the teacher responds to class participation and then often decide whether to risk exposing themselves by participating. The teacher who wishes to create a supportive atmosphere in which all students, including those who are culturally diverse, feel free to share their experiences must strive to reinforce and empower students when they contribute to class discussion.

Racial and cultural conflicts are difficult to deal with in groups. They require risking on an affective level and much self-awareness and support from everyone. These incidents in the classroom, however, are critical choice teaching points, because they provide on-the-spot opportunities to help students be open to these issues, as the following examples illustrate:

> In a class on supervision, an African-American supervisor presented a case involving a "difficult" employee. Students and the instructor provided numerous suggestions. For 15 minutes no one asked if the supervisee was from a different race (i.e., Caucasian). The instructor raised this. At first the class did not see the connection. The discussion changed, however. A West Indian student shared that she felt isolated from other African-American employees when she was promoted. A Haitian woman talked about her feelings of disgust when a Caucasian colleague spoke critically about Haitians. She was tired, however, of being a spokesperson and chose not to reveal her identity. The help given to the supervisor became more intense and meaningful. Group discussion in this area served to sensitize students to their own feelings about racial and power differences in agency practice as well as the larger community.

> * * * *

> In a group work class, a student presented his group of persons with AIDS, which he co-led. One student asked pejorative questions about AIDS and homosexuality. The class became very silent. Someone tried to divert the student asking questions. The presenting student asked the questioning student if she knew a person with AIDS. There was a deadening silence, as some of his classmates knew that the student presenting was

HIV positive. The instructor opened up discussion about AIDS and oppressed populations, which led to interactive learning over the hearing of a case study.

IMPACT OF AUTHORITY

A crucial beginning issue in all groups is working with authority issues (Shulman, 1992). After the teacher has handled the first student question of "what are we here for," the second central question is "what kind of person will the worker (teacher) be?" In all groups, members try to "size up" the authority figure as soon as possible (Shulman, 1992). The importance of the teachers' appropriate use of authority in the classroom has been stressed. "How teachers carry out their own authority–what they actually do–may make an even more important impact upon students than what they actually teach about authority" (Kurland, 1991, p. 84).

Just as group members may challenge the authority of the leader, so do students test out the teacher directly and indirectly. Often this is done by informal student leaders, and the educator may find it very threatening. These self-selected group leaders are frequently, but not always, from the white middle class majority, and their presence may also be threatening to the culturally diverse students. It has been noted that Caucasian students often emerge as class leaders, while persons of color often retreat to the back of the classroom and are less assertive (Gitterman, 1991). The teacher must strive to listen to all voices within the classroom, not only the informal group leaders. A frequent criticism of faculty on student evaluations is that certain students seem to dominate class discussion and receive encouragement in this from the teacher.

The social work educator should not automatically assume that student silence means acceptance of the teacher's authority. Just as client silence in social work practice can mean anger or fear (Kadushin, 1990; Shulman, 1992), student silence may indicate distrust of the social work educator. This may be particularly true of culturally diverse students who have often been oppressed within the white-dominated educational system (Pinderhughes, 1989). There may be a great deal of mistrust of white authority figures on the part of African-American students in graduate schools (Gitterman, 1991).

The teacher must try to work through authority issues with all class members. Social work teachers should not be authoritarian, but they definitely are authorities and have power and influence because of their role, position, and knowledge (Kurland, 1991). Also, the importance of strong leadership at the beginning of group sessions has been stressed (Shulman, 1992).

The following example illustrates a social work educator's attempt to deal with power and racial issues that emerge in the classroom:

> A group work class participating in a joint activity had formed several subgroups. All but one of the subgroups were culturally diverse. Near the end of the exercise the nondiverse, Caucasian group placed its production on top of the other groups. The other groups expressed their anger and in the midst of the conflict an African-American man stated that "maybe we ought to be dealing with tolerance." This comment was ignored until the instructor said, "Let's go back to Ray's comment and deal with this from that moment." The instructor pointed out some of the differences in the groups by sharing her own feelings.

To facilitate opening up discussion and participation among all class members, teachers need to be open to self-disclosing about their own feelings, as well as their practice experiences and educational background. Sometimes the educator's sharing will promote students' willingness to discuss culturally sensitive issues.

WORKING WITH THE INDIVIDUAL AND THE GROUP

An essential, but often challenging, issue in group work is working with the individuals in the group as well as the group as a whole (Schwartz, 1976). If the social worker fails to work with these two clients simultaneously, there is often a danger of perpetuating scapegoating (Shulman, 1992). Often social workers, because of their concern for social justice, try to support the scapegoat and doing this may prevent the group members from becoming further involved.

The difficulties of working with the individual as well as the group are particularly challenging in social work education. Social work students come from diversified educational, experiential, and cultural backgrounds. Often the student who is somewhat different from the majority of students may run the risk of being scape-goated, as the following example indicates:

> One culturally diverse student, who had limited educational experiences, participated in class discussion by describing at length cases from her child welfare practice. Initially, the teacher did not tune in that this student was becoming the class scapegoat. When this student began to talk other students would to roll their eyes, look though their books, or take a break. The teacher, concerned that this student would feel rejected, was always sure to reinforce positively what she said. The behavior of others became even more distracting.

As in the previous example, often the social work educator's position is to support students who are scapegoated. These students may have had previous negative experiences in negotiating an educational system in which they were different. By supporting the scapegoat, however, the teacher found that the class as a whole had become more distant and removed. Applying group work skills of working with the group as well as the individual, the social work educator could have reached for the commonality of this student's experience by asking if other students, especially those in child welfare, had had similar experiences. Also, in working with this individual student, the educator could have helped her explore new ways of looking at her experiential material, and connecting her practice experience with theory (Gitterman, 1991).

NEGOTIATING CONFLICT

Unfortunately, racial and ethnic tensions and conflict are com-mon in our society, and social work education is not immune from these issues. Social workers may often be unaware of their own biases and their responsibility in perpetuating an "us and them" dichotomy. This dichotomy is often seen at the root of racial and ethnic conflict (Lum, 1992). The classroom can be used to break down this false dichotomy, as the following examples demonstrate:

A clinical practice class enacted a role play about a battered women's group. The subgroup included four African-American women, a Latino woman, and one Caucasian woman. In the context of the activity, one African-American woman presented herself as a wealthy upper-middle-class woman. Her classmates began laughing and teasing her. "Get off it!" "What are you doing?" She defended herself and said that battered women occur in all classes. The subgroup and other class members continued to tease her. One Caucasian woman dressed in business attire shared that she was battered and that the African-American woman was portraying a real character. The instructor then halted the process to allow the group to look at itself and why they had difficulty accepting the role play.

* * * *

In a course on how systems affect direct practice, a student raised this issue. A university which wanted to increase Latino admissions took in a group of students with poorer academic credentials than its Caucasian mainstream body. As a result, 30 percent of its Latino population were brought to the Academic Committee with the outcome unfavorable to the students. The Latino students were not prepared for the academic review process. They were unable to present a clear defense or did not know how to use peer counseling or other resource networks. The student presenting this to the class stated that if there were concern about admitting people of color, there must be a commitment to getting them through. The professor felt quite anxious, but immediately asked for class involvement. A lively and difficult discussion followed. One African-American student stated he only goes to Caucasian doctors because of the "equal opportunity garbage." Another Latino student commented that she would not want people of her cultural background underserved by a less than adequate social worker. An older Caucasian student talked about her difficulties in returning to school and the fact that no one gave her extra support. The discussion finally moved to whether the dominant culture was responsible for diverse students' difficulties or were the students just not able to handle a graduate curriculum. Intervention strategies were developed and a decision was made to hold a panel presentation with a possible outcome being a strategy to approach the university.

These examples provided opportunities for the teacher to discuss cultural and racial biases which need to be identified in order to reduce conflict. Even when this conflict is unspoken, the social work educator must be aware of these differences and make the unspoken but divisive conflicts more open. This has been seen as an important use of the classroom group in social work education (Adams and Schlesinger, 1988). Just as in work with families, social workers must examine their own values and how this impacts on their work (Aponte, 1991); also, educators must examine their own values in preparation for work with diverse students.

Some issues of conflict which have arisen in social work classes with religiously and culturally diverse students include abortion, affirmative action, and kinship placements. It is essential that the social work educator acknowledge all voices in discussing these and other controversial issues, despite the social work educator's own personal and professional beliefs. One pro-life clergyman once told his students that they were aware of his beliefs about abortion, but he felt that the diversity of opinions on this issue was something he felt they could and should discuss within the classroom. Often the culturally diverse student who is a numerical minority within the classroom and has a dissenting opinion may be reluctant to speak unless encouraged by the teacher. The social work educator must serve as a model for encouraging and respecting the expression of diverse viewpoints.

BUILDING RELATIONSHIPS AND COALITIONS

An important task in group work is to build a cohesive group and this is often achieved through the development of mutual support in groups (Gitterman and Shulman, 1986). Often, within the classroom, different subgroups of culturally diverse students may develop. The social work educator notices these groupings in classroom seating as well as during breaks and at lunch. Mutual support may exist within these groups (Egan and Bombyk, 1991), but there may not be any mutual support between groups of ethnically and racially diverse students. The social work educator may want to encourage relationships and coalitions between and among diverse students.

This process can be facilitated both in daily class interaction as well as through class assignments. One way to facilitate classroom connections of diverse students is through pointing out similarities in experiences, as in the following example:

> A black Haitian social work student shared a case example from her agency child welfare practice. The teacher then connected this student with a white upper-middle-class student who also worked in child welfare by turning to this student and asking if the second student had had a similar experience with a foster parent.

The use of subgroups for social work assignments has been seen as an important learning tool in social work education (Latting and Raffoul, 1991). An additional benefit of group assignments is to encourage culturally diverse students to work cooperatively with other students from different backgrounds. Although at times the social work educator may want students to self-determine in choosing a group for completing an assignment, subgroups which develop are often racially and ethnically similar. To facilitate the formation of subgroups which bridge cultural differences, the social work educator may want to assign students to groups based on similar work experiences. Through participation in group learning assignments, diverse students are often able to form connections that may extend beyond the limits of the class assignments.

CONCLUSIONS AND RECOMMENDATIONS

Classroom teaching emerges as a powerful mechanism for increasing cultural sensitivity. This is true not only in classes that focus specifically on cultural diversity, but throughout the social work curriculum. To promote social work's commitment to social justice and antidiscrimination, social work educators can use group work skills to achieve these objectives. Students may learn more from what they experience in the classroom than from what they are taught didactically about cultural diversity.

Racial and cultural conflicts are difficult to deal with in groups. Opening up discussion in these areas involves risk-taking and greater self-awareness on the part of social work educators. These critical incidents provide opportunity for the teacher to use group process in helping students increase cultural sensitivity.

To facilitate the use of the classroom to model and promote cultural sensitivity in social work students, the following recommendations have been developed:

1. Social work educators must assess and understand their own beliefs, assumptions, and misconceptions about culturally diverse students and clients. Social work educators often come from backgrounds that may not be very accepting of cultural differences. We all live in a society where there are many biases and prejudices about people who are different. To teach more effectively, teachers must become more aware of how their attitudes influence their teaching about culturally diverse clients and to culturally diverse students.

2. Social work educators need to become more aware of their power as role models to their students. While it is important is what they tell students about being sensitive to cultural differences, even more crucial is what educators demonstrate in classrooms about acceptance and empowerment of diverse students.

3. Social work educators can use group work skills in promoting cultural sensitivity within the classroom. Many social work faculty come to educational institutions from a casework background. As teachers, however, they quickly learn the importance of group work skills in conducting a class. To be effective teachers, social work educators must continually strive to improve their group work skills.

4. Classes throughout the social work curriculum can be used to increase the cultural sensitivity of students. This can be accomplished by facilitating discussions on controversial issues and promoting intercultural collaboration. To create a culturally sensitive learning environment, the student must be allowed and encouraged to take risks. By promoting cultural sensitivity within the classroom, it is hoped that student awareness of

themselves, each other, their clients, and the larger community will be increased.

REFERENCES

Adams, A. and Schlesinger, E. (1988). Group approach to training ethnic-sensitive practitioners. In C. Jacobs and D. Bowles (eds.) *Ethnicity and race: Critical concepts in social work.* Silver Springs, MD: NASW.

Aponte, H. (1991). Training of the person of the therapist for work with the poor and minorities. *Journal of Independent Social Work 7*(3/4), 23-39.

Brown, L. (1991). *Groups for growth and change.* New York: Longman Publishers.

Chau, K. (1990). A model for teaching cross-cultural practice in social work. *Journal of Social Work Education 26*(2), 124-133.

_____ . (1991). Introduction: Facilitating bicultural development and intercultural skills in ethnically heterogenous groups. In R. Chau (ed.), *Ethnicity and biculturalism: Emerging perspectives of social group work.* New York: The Haworth Press, Inc.

Congress, E. (1992). Ethical teaching of multicultural students: Reconsideration of social work values for educators. *Journal of Multicultural Social Work 2*(2), 11-23.

Council on Social Work Education (1990). *Statistics on social work education in the United States, 1989.* Alexandria, VA: Council on Social Work Education.

Davis, L. and Proctor, E. (1989). *Race, gender, and class: Guidelines for practice with individuals, families, and groups.* Englewood Cliffs, NJ: Prentice Hall.

Egan, S. and Bombyk, M. (1991, March). *Multicultural dimensions of the third shift: Employed students who are mothers.* Paper presented at the Annual Program Meeting, Council on Social Work Education, New Orleans, LA.

Gitterman, A. (1991). Working with difference: White teacher and African-American students. *Journal of Teaching in Social Work 5*(2), 65-78.

Gitterman, A. and Shulman, L. (1986). *Mutual aid groups and the life cycle.* Itasca, IL: Peacock Publishers.

Glassman, U. (1991). Teaching ethno-racial sensitivity through groups. In K. Chau (ed.), *Ethnicity and biculturalism: Emerging perspectives of social group work.* New York: The Haworth Press, Inc.

Guttierez, L. and Ortega, R. (1991). Developing methods to empower Latinos: The importance of groups. *Social Work with Groups 14*(2), 23-43.

Kadushin, A. (1992). *Supervision in social work* (3rd ed.). New York: Columbia University Press.

_____ . (1990). *The social work interview* (3rd ed.). New York: Columbia University Press.

Kurland, R. (1991). The classroom teacher and the role of authority. *Journal of Teaching in Social Work 5*(2), 81-94.

Latting, J. (1990). Identifying the "isms": Enabling socialwork students to confront their biases. *Journal of Social Work Education. 26(3),* 36-44.

Latting, J. and Raffoul P. (1991). Designing student work groups for increased learning: An empirical investigation. *Journal of Social Work Education 27*(1), 48-59.

Lewis, H. (1987). Teaching ethnics through ethical teaching. *Journal of Teaching in Social Work 1*(1), 3-14.

_____ . (1991). Teacher's style and use of professional self in social work education. *Journal of Teaching in Social Work 5*(2), 17-29.

Lewis, E. and Ford, B. (1991). The network utilization project: Incorporating traditional strengths of African American families into group work practice. In K. Chau (ed.). *Ethnicity and biculturalism: Emerging perspectives of social group work.* New York: The Haworth Press, Inc.

Lum, D. (1992). *Social work practice and people of color: A process-stage approach.* (2nd ed.). Pacific Grove, CA: Brooks Cole.

Manoleas, P. and Carrillo, E. (1991). A culturally syntonic approach to the field education of Latino students. *Journal of Social Work Education, 27*(2), 135-144.

McGoldrick, M., Pearce, J. and Giordano, J. (eds.) (1982). *Ethnicity and family therapy.* New York: Guilford Press.

Norman, A. (1991). The use of the group and group work techniques in resolving interethnic conflict. *Social Work with Groups, 14*(3/4), 175-186.

Oliver, J. and Brown, L. (1988). The development and implementation of a minority recruitment plan: Process, strategy, and results. *Journal of Social Work Education 24*(2), 175-185.

Pinderhughes, E. (1989). *Understanding race, ethnicity, and power.* New York: The Free Press.

Schwartz, W. (1964). The classroom teaching of social work with groups. In *A conceptual framework for the teaching of the social group work method in classroom.* New York: Council on Social Work Education.

_____ . (1976). Between client and system: The mediating function. In R. Roberts and H. Northen (eds.), *Theories of social work with groups.* New York: Columbia University Press.

Shulman, L. (1987). The hidden group in the classroom: The use of group process in teaching group work practice. *Journal of Teaching in Social Work 1*(2), 3-31.

_____ . (1992). *The skills of helping individuals, families, and groups.* Itasca, IL: Peacock Publisher.

Solomon, B. (1976). *Black empowerment.* New York: Columbia University Press.

Yalom, I. (1988). *The theory and practice of group psychotherapy.* New York: Basic Books.

Chapter 8

Towards Mutual Aid in Groups: Issues in a Chinese Society

Fanny W. C. L. Liu

As an international city, Hong Kong is affected by values from different ethnic groups, especially from Britain and America. Likewise social work practice and education have also been imported from Britain and America and adopted for use locally. Despite the demand for indigenous materials in the 1960s, it is only in the last decade that more local writing has emerged. For example, a book on *Group Work Practice* (Ng et al., 1992) was prepared and incorporated reflections on the application of group work models in the local context. Pearson (1991) addressed particularly the cultural issues in group work practice and pointed out some of the incompatibilities between Western theories and the Eastern practice of group work.

Being such a dynamic city, it is difficult to conclude whether Hong Kong is upholding the traditional Chinese values or submitting to the influence of Western culture (Bond, 1986). It may be more feasible to explore the cultural compatibility by choosing a more focused theme. In this paper, mutual aid is chosen as an entry point for the inquiry.

MUTUAL AID IN GROUPS

Peter Kropotkin (1916), in his classic *Mutual Aid*, emphasized the power of mutual aid as a factor in cultural and social evolution by recording a number of impressive facts. The late William Schwartz (1961), who was the pioneer of the interactionist approach, declared that the focal point of a worker's intervention should be on fostering mutual aid among clients and workers, and within the general society. He stated that,

> The group is an enterprise in mutual aid, an alliance of individuals who need each other, in varying degrees, to work on certain common problems. The important fact is that this is a helping system in which the clients need each other as well as the worker. This need to use each other, to create not one but many helping relationships, is a vital ingredient of the group process and constitutes a common need over and above the specific tasks for which the group was formed. (p. 18)

A similar notion is evident in major writing on social work with groups. For instance, Papell and Rothman (1980) referred to a group as a potential mutual aid system; Hartford (1976:49) regarded a group as a helping context in which the individual, aided by the social support of other members, could gain self-understanding; and McBroom (1976:271) suggested that a group was a promoter of mutual responsibilities. In the process of distilling and identifying the central theme of group work, Papell and Rothman, referred to earlier, stated that the mainstream group was characterized by common goals, mutual aid, and nonsynthetic experiences, and they declared that the conception of the group as a mutual aid system had become universal in group work practice. Thus, the achievement of mutual aid became an indicator of success for social work groups.[1]

In reviewing writing on mutual aid in groups, some basic features can be concluded about the group itself, about the group members, and about the group leader.

The Group Itself

The group members share common problems or common experience. Because of the need for one another, different kinds of helping relationships can be formed. Lenneberg and Rowbotham (1970) stated that the essence of mutual help was exchange. Therefore, a mutual aid group should allow space and opportunities for sharing, not only among members but between the worker and the members.

Lee and Swenson (1986:371) maintained that the "concept of forming groups around shared experiences can, of course, be applied in any setting, with any population sharing a common situation." In other words, a group of people sharing a common concern is potentially a mutual aid group.

The Group Members

To achieve mutual aid, each member in a group has certain obligations toward his fellow members, and perhaps particularly in Hong Kong where the lack of democratic practice in an organizational context may have both a direct and indirect effect on mutual aid in groups. The participant is expected to show concern about the condition and progress of other members, and to provide them with support, acceptance, and opportunities to experiment. The underlying faith is on the ability of the client not only to help himself/herself, but also to help others. In a group, the members reach out for each other to render help.

Riessman (1965) suggested that it could be helpful for a person to be a helper. Skovholt (1974) further elaborated on the "helper therapy" principle and summarized that in being an effective helper, one may have a higher level of interpersonal competence; feel a sense of equality in giving and taking; receive a valuable, personalized experience while helping others; and receive social approval from those who are helped. In this sense, members in mutual aid groups are expected to become actively involved in the process and to be reinforced by taking actions to support others.

The Group Leader

In signifying the importance of the function of leader, Shulman (1979) remarked that "the potential for mutual aid exists in the group; simply bringing people together does not guarantee that it will emerge." Tropp (1976) highlighted the role of a worker in fostering a supportive environment in which members could develop their own mutual aid system. The worker was herself a caring and respectable model who facilitated a sense of connection in the group. Wasserman and Danforth (1988) summarized the functions of a group leader as being

> to encourage and model information sharing; mediate differing opinions; give permission to discuss taboo areas and emphasize the common bond; reinforce and demonstrate empathic responses and build mutual support; support mutual demands while validating the expectations for all members to work; allow individual problem solving and help group members to assume consultant role; and, engage members in a rehearsal of behaviors. (p. 143)

Conclusively, a group having members sharing common concerns provides a basis for developing mutual aid. The reciprocal helping relationship is not limited to members, but extends to include the worker. Thus, the functions of the worker in fostering mutual aid are modeling, mediating, and performing skills so as to develop a group culture.

CULTURAL FACTORS IN HONG KONG

In the process of promoting mutual aid in groups in Hong Kong, it is not surprising that workers encounter obstacles similar to those highlighted by the American theorists. For example, the inability of some group members to identify with the pain and suffering of others; the general failure in group development; the difficulty in establishing the norm of honest communication; and a group leader's lack of awareness or interest in mutual aid as a high human value (Wasserman and Danforth, 1988:145). Nevertheless, the cultural heritage of Hong Kong provides a different ground to test out this Western concept. To some extent, cultural factors can facilitate or hinder the development of mutual aid in groups.

The Effect of the Traditional Chinese Heritage

As a metropolitan city where people from different parts of the world will meet, and as one of the financial centers in the world, it is undeniable that Hong Kong is capitalistic in nature. Together with the strong emphasis on using English as a medium of education, it seems reasonable to say that the people of Hong Kong are inclined to accept the western value of individualism. Nevertheless, this view is not totally supported by research findings. For example, Lau (1981) found that Chinese people in Hong Kong were still very familistic. Chan (1986) and Wong (1986) concluded that deep inside the mind of Hong Kong people, they still cling to some of the traditional Chinese values and are motivated by various aspects of social living.

The Chinese Culture

In Chinese culture, man is a social relational being. He is socially situated and defined within an interactive context (Bond, 1986). The five cardinal relations (*wu lu*) guide Chinese people to act according to their location in the interactive context. It is believed that harmony would be realized if each member of the unit were conscientious in following the expected role performance. The rules of correct behavior (*li*) entail both rights and responsibilities for each role. While *li* guides a person to behave properly, humanism (*ren*) denotes a bilateral relationship inferring interdependency among people.

Yang (1981) recalled Confucius' emphasis on interrelatedness and concluded that Chinese people tended "to submit to social expectations, social conformity, . . . in a social situation." He considered that modern Chinese people might give greater weight to their own personal standards, but they were still attached to the anticipated reactions of others to their behavior. The interplay of *face (lien), reciprocation (bao), and relationship (guanxi)* in Chinese culture (Hwang, 1983) further maintains the cohesion of a group, though the group may not be functioning toward mutual aid.

Chinese are regarded as collectivists. A study by Gabrenya and Wang (1983) found that Chinese men and women were more likely to endorse group-oriented self-concepts than were Americans. A collectivized culture emphasizes the importance of maintaining the integrity of groups against the diverse forces of self-interest. Thus, a person's degree of conscientiousness is closely tied to his/her responsibility toward others during interactions. Submission to comments from others may reinforce *li* and conformity to reference groups.

Li guides a person to behave according to a role expectation. *Ren* emphasizes the duty of reciprocal relationships. Interrelatedness is a central precept of Chinese people who have submitted to social expectations, reflecting the importance of maintaining group integrity in Chinese heritage. These characteristics seem to form a basis for using groups as an effective tool. The same factors, however, may be used for controlling purposes or for facilitating mutual aid. This is a particularly sensitive issue in a society such as Hong Kong that has a long history of being governed by a colonial government and has not experienced much liberalization of human rights. The impact of these factors in enhancing or hindering the development of mutual aid in groups will be explored further.

Impact on Groups

For a group to have the potential to develop mutual aid, the members need to share common concerns. Through sharing and mutual exchange, helping relationships can be formed. In a Chinese society, such as in Hong Kong, some cultural factors may be a hindrance to the development of such relationships in a group.

The hierarchical structure predetermines the role and role-related social behaviors. For Chinese people, the disclosure of personal matters is thus limited to those of expressive ties.[2] In mixed ties, such as in a social work group, it is impossible for members to disclose themselves, especially at an early stage. Chinese norms tend to treasure harmony. For the sake of the maintenance of harmony, the discrepancy between public presentation and private belief is relatively great (Bond, 1986:257). The individual's actual position on an issue is subordinated to his/her desire to protect the group's integrity by side-stepping open disagreement (Wilson, 1974). The priority given to the family as the locus of sharing deep feelings and personal matters (Goffman, 1967) and the tendency to treasure group integrity more than personal freedom of choice may further stop members from revealing and opening up themselves.

The reciprocal nature of *ren* is perceived as the duty or responsibility of a man to another man. This is different from the voluntary and genuine nature of giving and receiving help in interpersonal relations in the Western culture. Subsequently, a reciprocal relationship may be perceived as a demand and burden to a member who tries hard to keep harmony and wants to be regarded as a conscientious person.

Another cultural factor is the perception of needs. Hong Kong Chinese do not generally seek professional help for mild emotional problems and when they do, they tend to approach a medical practitioner (Cheung, Lee, and Chan, 1983). Chinese people tend to accept physical sickness more than psychological difficulties. This is often manifested in their attitudes toward mental illness. This way of perceiving needs will limit the scope of sharing to discussions of physical complaints, rather than of personal and inner feelings.

Impact on Group Members

To create mutual aid, group members are expected to be active, open, and involved in being a helper. These qualities differ from the Chinese mode to a great extent.

In a study of personal traits, Chang (1983) summarized that the most frequently mentioned traits of Chinese students were being humble, altruistic, honest, hard-working, generous, and graceful in speech. This can reflect the expectation of self and others in interpersonal relationships. In mixed ties, as in a group, members may act in accordance with their social idea. As a result of being humble, active involvement of Chinese group members is not apparent. Coupled with the restrained emotional expression of Chinese people, it is difficult for them to initiate a sharing of their feelings among the members. Moreover, exposing a person's mistake may provoke public reaction and create disharmony. Chinese people usually show a heightened reluctance to criticize others.

To achieve mutual aid, group members need to be open. In this way, different opinions will be raised. Face-saving has minimized the chance of open conflict. Even in conflicting situations, Chinese strategies for resolving these conflicts are characterized by the use of indirect language, a middleman, flexibility, and so on (Hwang, 1978). Direct confrontation is avoided (Bond et al., 1985).

When confronted with crisis, Hwang (1978) identified five strategies of Chinese coping.[3] The most frequent coping responses of Hong Kong Chinese people, irrespective of the nature of the problems (Shek and Mak, 1987), are the mobilization of personal resources and a philosophy of doing nothing. The former strategy includes the mechanism of face reality and self-assertion. Hwang (1978) found that when Chinese people used much self-assertion, they tended to attribute this to the fault of others. Regarding the choice of coping strategies, there are two implications for members' behavior. First, the use of a doing-nothing strategy and self-assertion by blaming others will minimize a member's contribution to solving the problems of others and to confronting his/her own problem. Second, the tendency of not seeking help from social resources indicates a resistance to seeking help from friends or from professionals.

Chang (1983) found that for Chinese students of both sexes , the affiliation tendency was positively related to self-perceived sociometric status and to self-evaluation. By being a helper instead of being in a sick role, members may have a higher self-evaluation and be in a better sociometric position in the group. Thus, there will be a higher level of group affiliation.

Based on the above influences, it seems that Chinese group members may be more hesitant and reluctant to become involved but, on the other hand, their involvement as helpers is likely to lead to the development of group coheshion.

Impact on the Group Leader and Leadership

Shulman (1979) has identified processes to enhance mutual aid in groups and the group leader as the key person to facilitate the development of mutual aid. In Hofstede's study (1983), examples were given that Chinese subjects have a highly collective profile and the need to be moderately high in power distance.[4] People in large power distance societies accept a hierarchical order in which everybody has a place which needs no further justification. This brings forth a number of considerations for group leaders seeking to enhance mutual aid.

First, in the Chinese games of face saving, one has to speak in the language suited to one's situation and display appropriate behavior and status symbols. Because of the need to save the face of the worker, who is normally regarded as being in a superior position, it seems impossible to build up an equal and reciprocal relationship between group worker and members.

Second, research findings (Meade, 1970; Bennett, 1977) have suggested that Chinese groups function smoothly with more authoritarian interaction patterns between superior and subordinate. Chinese groups were more cohesive when they had a controlling style of leadership, and a task-oriented leader was regarded as a more efficient leader. There is a similar phenomenon in group work practice in Hong Kong. In the writer's experience, members prefer a leader who can maintain a harmonious, considerate relationship with the members, but he/she should also be able to take skilled and decisive actions. To a certain extent, this contradicts the worker's main function, (which is to mediate rather than to "cure") in developing mutual aid.

Third, a worker who is also Chinese may be affected by the need to preserve the face of members and his/her own as well. The worker may be reluctant to open up himself/herself, especially when his/her status of being an expert is threatened. He/she may be afraid of being rejected by the group members. He/she also may feel shameful of declaring his or her fear, and so on. Therefore, it is crucial for the worker to accept his/her own limitations and thus to disclose himself/herself in an appropriate manner and situation.

Fourth, Hong Kong Chinese people do not often seek help from social resources. Even when they seek help from social resources, friends and parents are more likely to be approached than professional help (Shek and Mak, 1987; Boys and Girls Clubs Association of Hong Kong, 1992). The leader thus can predict some sort of resistance from the members in receiving service from professionally led groups. Passive resistance is commonly encountered. On the other hand, the members may be so desperate that they have given up hope. Thus, they will demand that the leader work for them and give instructions as a doctor does. The self-expected role of members of being passive and sick versus active offers a challenge for leaders in cultivating an open and supportive group culture.

Fifth, Chinese people expect their leader to have the power of anticipating and diffusing potential confrontations among members. The leader should take immediate action to terminate the encounter and to smooth over the issue in private before another meeting takes place (Bond et al., 1985). This performance expectation of the leader differs greatly from that of a mutual aid group. Members resist being open, even in conflicting situations, and they expect the group leader to intervene in order to avoid conflict.

The function of a group leader is vital in facilitating the development of mutual aid. It is more important in a Chinese society because of the reasons stated above. In practicing group work, members usually have dual expectations of the leader. On the one hand, they want the group to be structured, leader-centered, and filled up with tasks. On the other hand, they expect the worker to be genuine, polite, member-centered, and to move at their pace. They are not willing to express their discontent in a group, but prefer to approach the leader after group sessions in order to protect themselves from being labeled as "deviant from the group." In interacting, they rely heavily on the worker for approval and agreement. Despite the background of the group members, they expect the worker to take the guiding and leading role. They may not necessarily be submissive to the authority of the leader and may even reject the suggestion of the leader in private, but still they regard the leader as someone who should bear all the responsibilities for the group.

The very nature of traditional Chinese heritage seems to form a nurturing ground for the use of groups for Chinese people. However, when mutual aid is to be developed in groups, cultural factors form obstacles to achieving such an end. A group worker who is the leader of a professionally led group will need to work through such resistance before mutual aid in groups in a Chinese society such as in Hong Kong can be feasible.

NOTES

1. Groups in this paper refer to professionally led, formed groups in social work practice.

2. Hwang (1983) classified interpersonal relationships in Chinese society into three main categories based on their expressive and instrumental components. They are expressive ties, instrumental ties, and mixed ties. Expressive ties are relationships between members in a family. Instrumental ties are relationships that an individual may establish temporarily and anonymously with other people solely as a means to attain his or her personal goals. Mixed ties are a kind of interpersonal relationship in which an individual is most likely to play a power game.

3. The five strategies of Chinese coping included mobilization of personal resources, seeking help from social resources, appealing to supernatural power, the doing-nothing philosophy, and other forms of avoidance.

4. Power distance is the extent to which the members of a society accept that power which is distributed unequally in institutions and organizations.

REFERENCES

Bennett, M. (1977). Testing Management Theories Cross Culturally, *Journal of Applied Social Psychology*, 62, pp. 578-81.

Bond, M., Wan, K. C., Leung, K., and Giacalone, R. (1985). How Are Responses to Verbal Insult Related to Cultural Collectivism and Power Distance? *Journal of Cross-Cultural Psychology*, 16, pp. 111-27.

Bond, M. (Ed.) (1986). *The Psychology of the Chinese People*, Hong Kong: Oxford.

Boys & Girls Clubs Association of Hong Kong (1992). *Help-Seeking Tendency of Young People in Hong Kong*, Hong Kong: Boys & Girls Clubs Association of Hong Kong.

Chan, P. (1986). A Multi-faceted Approach for Young Social Workers in Working with Chinese Families in Hong Kong, *Hong Kong Journal of Social Work*, 20/2, pp. 13-19.

Chang, W. J. (1983). Affiliation Tendency and Sociometric Status, *Bulletin of Educational Psychology*, 13, pp. 153-78. (In Chinese)

Cheung, F. M., Lee, S. Y. & Chan, Y. Y. (1983). Variations in Problem Conceptualizations and Intended Solutions Among Hong Kong Students, *Culture, Medicine and Psychiatry*, 7, pp. 263-78.

Gabrenya, W. K. & Wang, Y. E. (1983). Cultural Differences in Self-Schemata: China and the United States. Paper presented at the meeting of the Southeast Psychological Association, Atlanta, GA.

Goffman, E. (1967). *Interaction Ritual*, New York: Doubleday.

Hartford, M. E. (1976). Group Methods and Generic Practice. In Roberts, R. & H. Northen (Eds.) *Theories of Social Work with Groups*, New York: Columbia University Press.

Hofstede, G. (1983). Dimensions of National Cultures in Fifty Countries and Three Regions. In Deregowski, J. B., Dzinrawiec, S. & R. C. Annis (Eds.) *Expiscations in Cross-cultural Psychology*, Netherlands: Swets & Zeithinger, pp. 335-55.

Hwang, K. (1978). The Dynamic Processes of Coping with Interpersonal Conflicts in a Chinese Society, *Proceedings of the National Science Council*, 2/2, pp. 198-208.

_____ . (1983). Face and Favor: Chinese Power Games, Unpublished manuscript, National Taiwan University.

Kropotkin, P. (1916). *Mutual Aid*, New York: Alfred Knopf.

Lau, S. K. (1981). Chinese Familism in an Urban-Industrial Setting: The Case of Hong Kong, *Journal of Marriage and the Family*, Vol. 43, No. 4, pp. 148-153.

Lee, J. & C. R. Swenson (1986). The Concept of Mutual Aid. In Gitterman, A. & L. Shulman (Eds.) *Mutual Aid Groups and the Life Cycle*, pp. 361-377.

Lenneberg, A. & Rowbotham, G. (1970). *The Ileostomy Patient*, Springfield, IL: C. Thomas.

Meade, R. D. (1970). Leadership Studies of Chinese and Chinese-Americans, *Journal of Cross-Cultural Psychology*, 1, pp. 325-32.

McBroom, E. (1976). Socialization Through Small Groups. In Roberts, R. & H. Northen (Eds.) *Theories of Social Work with Groups*, New York: Columbia University Press, pp. 268-303.

Ng, A., Au, C. F., Au, C. K., Chan, A., Choi, K.W., and Choi, P. K. (Eds.) (1992). *Group Work Practice*, Hong Kong: Hong Kong Social Workers' Association. (In Chinese).

Papell, C. & B. Rothman (1980). Relating the Mainstream Model of Social Work with Groups to Group Psychotherapy and the Structural Group Approach, *Social Work with Groups*, 3/2, pp. 5-23.

Pearson, V. (1991). Western Theory, Eastern Practice: Social Group Work in Hong Kong, *Social Work with Groups*, 14/2, pp. 45-58.

Riessman, F. (1965). The Helper's Therapy Principle, *Social Work*, 10, pp. 27-32.

Schwartz, W. (1961). The Social Worker in the Group. In *New Perspectives on Services to Groups*, New York: National Association of Social Workers, pp. 7-34.

Shek, D. & J. Mak (1987). *Psychological Well-Being of Working Parents in Hong Kong: Mental Health, Stress and Coping Responses*, Hong Kong: Hong Kong Christian Service.

Shulman, L. (1979). *The Skills of Helping Individuals and Groups*, Itasca, IL: F. E. Peacock.

Skovholt, T. M. (1974). The Client as Helper: A Means to Promote Psychological Growth, *Counselling Psychologist*, 4/3, pp. 58-64.

Tropp, E. (1976). A Developmental Theory. In Roberts, R. & H. Northen (Eds.) *Theories of Social Work with Groups*, New York: Columbia University Press, pp. 198-237.

Wasserman, H. & H. Danforth (1988). *The Human Bond: Support Groups and Mutual Aid*, New York: Springer Publishing Co.

Wilson, R. W. (1974). *The Moral State: A Study of the Political Socialization of Chinese and American Children*, New York: The Free Press.

Wong, S. L. (1986). Modernization and Chinese Culture in Hong Kong, *The China Quarterly*, 106, pp. 306-325.

Yang, K. S. (1981). Social Orientation and Individual Modernity Among Chinese Students in Taiwan, *Journal of Social Psychology*, 113, pp. 159-70.

Chapter 9

Making Changes and Making Sense: Social Work Group with Vietnamese Older People

Paule McNicoll
Carole Pigler Christensen

THE CONTEXT

In recent years, schools of social work in Canada have been called upon to implement changes in their curricula which reflect multicultural and multiracial realities (Canadian Association of Schools of Social Work, 1991). A project to link schools of social work more closely to populations that often perceive a lack of access to social services was funded by Multiculturalism and Citizenship Canada. The Multicultural Family Center was created as part of this effort.

The social work group program with Vietnamese older people was the first undertaking of the Multicultural Family Center, a social service agency in a multiethnic neighborhood of Vancouver, British Columbia, Canada. The agency itself represents a joint venture of the School of Social Work at the University of British Columbia and REACH Community Health Center, a medical, dental, and preventive health facility. The mission of the Multicultural Family Center is to provide a field training site for students by offering selected social services to cultural communities, and to

The authors are grateful to the Ministry of Multiculturalism and Citizenship for the research funds that made this study possible. Dr. Christensen was the Principal Investigator.

disseminate knowledge based on the experience of learning to provide cross-cultural services. The creation of the Multicultural Family Center was preceded by a needs assessment survey (McNicoll and Christensen, 1993a) which uncovered the health and social needs of the Vietnamese elderly. The first project of the new center therefore aimed at serving this neglected population.

THE POPULATION

Older people from minority cultures are known to experience "double jeopardy" (Dowd and Bengston, 1978); in the case of the Vietnamese, one could use the term "multiple jeopardy." In addition to facing the usual adjustments associated with later life, the Vietnamese elderly have to come to terms with the loss of their country, the trauma of war and dislocation, the challenges of a new culture, a new language, and a new climate (Bernier, 1992; Dorais, Pilon-Le, and Nguyen, 1987). Moreover, older ethnic people are often forgotten, since younger adults are more visible (Gelfand, 1986; Lee, 1987) and are expected to have a greater economic impact on their new country.

In 1991, we conducted a needs assessment among professionals who work with the Vietnamese community (McNicoll and Christensen, 1993a). The results of this survey corroborated previous research findings which indicated that: Vietnamese older people experience social isolation (Cox, 1982), loss of status (Dorais, Pilon-Le, and Nguyen, 1987; Ruthledge, 1992), economic dependency on their children (Canadian Task Force on Mental Health Issues Affecting Immigrants and Refugees, 1988), and intergenerational conflicts (Alcohol/Drug Education Service, 1989; Chin, 1983). These seniors are at particular risk for depression and other mental health problems (Canadian Task Force on Mental Health Issues Affecting Immigrants and Refugees, 1988).

The respondents to our survey noted that Vietnamese seniors need counseling services, but, because of fear of stigma and unfamiliarity with "talking" therapies, it was unlikely that they would use such services. Furthermore, because most recent Vietnamese immigrants are not fluent in English, counseling would have to be offered by bilingual, bicultural professionals. Respondents suggested that the workers subscribe to the following criteria: high-quality service, cultural sensitivity, high ethical standards, and political neutrality. In order to use the service, moreover, many clients would need assistance with transportation fees.

LESSONS FROM THE LITERATURE

Although the literature dealing specifically with group work with elderly Vietnamese clients is limited, there is a growing body of literature dealing with groups among refugees, and the refugee experience generally (*Canadian Journal of Community Mental Health*, 1993; *Canadian Social Work Review*, 1991; *Journal of Multicultural Social Work*, 1992). During the implementation phase of the Multicultural Family Center, we had already taken into account four essential characteristics for agencies serving elderly clients from Asian cultures (Lee, Patchner, and Balgopal, 1991; McNicoll and Christensen, 1993b). These are: central location of the agency; staff and board members from the Asian culture to be served; special outreach efforts; and bicultural and bilingual staff. To meet the unique needs of the Vietnamese older people, we consulted the literature on: groups with the Vietnamese, people of Asian ancestry, older people, and immigrants and refugees.

Several authors recommend therapy groups for people who have been traumatized (Tribe and Shackman, 1989). Others emphasize that support and ESL may need to be combined (Tannenbaum, 1990). Gardella (1985) and Wong (1991) introduced group reminiscence in their work with elders. An experience of such group reminiscence with Jewish immigrants was documented by Myerhoff (1978), who concluded that the sharing of life stories had helped clients both socially and psychologically. Group facilitators who work with refugees also must take into consideration their clients' needs for education, support, community, and empowerment (Glassman and Skolnik, 1984). A study by Christensen (1985) indicated that prospective Chinese immigrant clients often lacked information about mainstream health and social services. But information is not always sufficient; clients may need some familiarity with the resources and some basic skills in order to access the services they need (Breton, 1985).

There are cautionary communications in the literature on groups with Asian people. Pearson (1991) reported that people from Hong Kong prefer a directive leader who makes decisions, acts as a teacher, and does not expect expression of emotions or self-disclosure. The Western belief in taking responsibility for one's fate conflicts with the passive receptivity of the Chinese (Pearson, 1991). Therefore, therapists must adapt their clinical styles to their clients' culture, focus on establishing a working alliance with these clients, and educate them about the purpose, process, and benefits of psychotherapy (Tsui and Schultz, 1985). The use of programmed activities is often a successful strategy to engage Asian clients (Chau, 1990).

ORIGINAL PLAN

The Multicultural Family Center devised a support group program for Vietnamese older people to meet their developmental, support, and language needs. The overall goals of the group program for the Vietnamese elderly were to: reduce social isolation, help them deal with loss and grief, support their coming to terms with their lives and history, increase their self-esteem and confidence, and increase their knowledge of English.

The original plan called for eight to 12 Vietnamese seniors to meet for one and a half hours once a week for a trial period of eight weeks to discuss issues about their present life and past history. The sessions were to be held in English with the possibility of speaking Vietnamese when someone's knowledge of English faltered. There was to be no translation during the group sessions and the facilitators were to encourage people to resume speaking English as soon as they could. The idea was for the two facilitators, a Vietnamese paraprofessional and a Canadian social worker, to introduce information and knowledge about local resources and services as specific needs were identified. The agency was to pay the public transportation expenses of those attending the group.

This format fit well with the request that we provide some form of counseling to the Vietnamese elders and with the constraints of our work situation: the limited space, the availability of only one Vietnamese-speaking facilitator, the supervisor's expertise with small group dynamics, the expectations of the social work trainees, and the Center's mandate of facilitating the integration of newcomers into Canadian society.

The format, however, was poorly received by the Vietnamese Advisory Committee, a local body composed of Vietnamese professionals and paraprofessionals in health and social services. They argued that the elders would not be able to communicate in English and would not like an approach that was unstructured and based on personal sharing. They suggested instead that we organize a large social group held in Vietnamese. Staff at the Multicultural Family Center took heed of these recommendations. We were able to meet the need for more structure and the need to work in Vietnamese. However, we decided to keep the small group format because our space was limited and we were uncertain of whether we could attract a strong following among the Vietnamese elderly. The Advisory Committee reinforced our resolve to be vigilant and flexible, and confirmed the importance of consulting with the community one hopes to serve at the planning stage.

THE FIRST GROUP PROGRAM

The group program was advertised in the Vietnamese media, and the Vietnamese facilitator asked other Vietnamese care providers for referrals. Eight Vietnamese elders, seven men and one woman, attended the first group meeting in April 1992. Few of them spoke English, and it was immediately obvious that this meeting and future ones had to be held in Vietnamese. After introductions were made and refreshments were served, the facilitators gave the participants a choice among many themes for the weeks to come. Group members assented to all themes, but were unwilling to express preferences. They left apparently satisfied and some spoke of bringing friends to the next meeting. Expecting a slight drop in attendance, the facilitators stated that the seniors were responsible for deciding what they wanted from their group and that a few friends would be welcome. The second week, there were 16 participants, the third week, 30. When the group had reached 40 members by the fifth week, some people had to sit on the floor. Still, group participants expressed satisfaction with the growth of the group. They stated that they felt more comfortable in a large crowd than in a more intimate setting. A bigger facility was needed.

The content of the sessions had to be changed, too. While the older people never rejected directly the notion of sharing their life stories, they did not appear to support it very strongly. By contrast, they showed much enthusiasm for special celebrations, field trips, and information on social resources, Canadian culture, housing, and health. These Vietnamese seniors voted with their feet and their smiles. From the second session on, the group program adopted a clear educational bent, in keeping with the wishes of the members; it included information about financial assistance, a tour of a nearby community center (approximately 30 members joined the community center on this occasion), a walk in the neighborhood, and lectures on medication, nutrition, and immigration procedures. The last session was a trip to Victoria, the capital of British Columbia, organized at the request of the seniors. At the end of each meeting, the facilitators made time for questions, discussion, and feedback. They also attended a weekly debriefing session with representatives of the School of Social Work and REACH Community Health Center.

The success of the group program alleviated our fear that it would take many months to attract seniors. The program was evaluated by a bilingual questionnaire during the eighth and last session of the first series of group sessions. Unfortunately, only 16 of the 43 seniors present responded.[1] All 16 indicated that the group was useful and convenient. They particularly liked the educational sessions, socializing, group discussions, field trips, the provision of bus tickets, and refreshments. No one indicated that there were any aspects of the program they disliked, but many were concerned about the size of the room (since the group has grown considerably), and some wanted more time for social interaction. Suggestions for the next series of group sessions included the desire for more information about health issues; information about services and benefits available to them; field trips; and opportunities to learn English and to exercise. Overall, comments indicated that the program was useful, that it needed to become permanent, and that the facilitators were most affable.

REVISED PROGRAM AND FORMAT

A local community center provided the group program with ideal facilities: a small kitchen, an office, and a huge living room. After a lull of two weeks, a new group program started in July 1992, devised to take into account the experience and the evaluation of the first series of group sessions. The goals of this program were to favor social interaction of the Vietnamese older people, promote their physical and mental health, empower them, and foster their integration into Canadian society. The new program would involve five hours, one day per week, for 20 consecutive weeks, and included an English class, gentle exercises, health screening, and a lecture followed by discussion on a topic of the clients' choice.

The two English classes were taught by a volunteer ESL teacher. As desired by the seniors, health was the main focus of study and practice conversation. The half-hour of gentle exercise was not only a means to encourage fitness, but also an opportunity for older people to experience one another in a different light. The exercise seemed to bring a touch of humor and relaxation to the otherwise formal atmosphere. The health screening consisted of short individual consultations with a health professional. This part of the program was criticized as being illness-centered by a local nurse active in the health promotion movement, but this person did not take into account that, for many years, health care had been neglected because Vietnamese people lacked resources and had to focus on immediate survival issues. For instance, during one screening of 11 seniors, an ophthalmologist discovered three people in immediate need of eye operations and five people who would see much better with glasses.

The lectures were quite varied, and focused on, for example: introductions to Canadian society (e.g., justice system, social welfare regulations, social assistance); health and well-being (e.g., high blood pressure, pet therapy); social problems (e.g., elder abuse, family violence); continuity of Vietnamese culture (e.g., Vietnam in 1993, consultation on the needs of the Vietnamese community in Vancouver); and existential issues (e.g., death and the meaning of life in different cultures). Once a month, there was either an outing (e.g., going to see a jury trial), a meeting with people of a different cultural background (e.g., fiesta with Latin-American elders, lunch with the Japanese, and a tea party with Canadian seniors), or a celebration (e.g., Moon Festival, Vietnamese New Year). Membership in this program was not limited, and most people who had attended the first group program became members of the following series. (See Figure 9.1.)

The effectiveness of the group was assessed by an independent evaluator (Fryer, 1992) who conducted focus groups with representatives of the seniors and interviews with key informants from the Vietnamese community. All six seniors involved in the focus groups were enthusiastic about the program. They said that the program was meeting their needs for socializing, information on resources, developing a sense of well-being, and mastery of their new environment. Examples of their comments follow (Fryer, 1992, p. 6):

> This is a good opportunity for us to meet people from the same country, to talk about happy things and sad things. Without the program, we wouldn't know where to go, we would just be at home with our children. When we first came here we didn't know the customs. We need to know more about Canada.

> Even if the location is small, you have created a common happiness for us. You can see this on everyone's face–that happiness. It's a chance to meet new friends, to understand about rules and regulations, and to learn about things like child abuse and elder abuse. We will know more as more workshops happen.

> Many of us have low self-esteem. We have lost everything. But we feel happy because of this program.

> This is an opportunity to meet many people. The facilitators are helpful. I feel happy when I come here, there are people to talk to. I didn't feel comfortable at first, but I feel comfortable now. All my family is away during the day–at work or at school.

> We have accumulated a lot. Martine and Lam treat us well. There are things we wanted to do, but didn't have the opportunity before. It's good that Lam and Martine have started the project since our children don't have time to take us places or answer our questions.

The participants attributed the success of the group to the respectful attitude and the competence of the group facilitators. They wanted the program to become more widely known and accessible. They suggested a heavier use of the Vietnamese media to publicize the group program. Some respondents also recommended the provision of childcare services, since many older people take care of their grandchildren during the day. Finally, one participant suggested that the seniors take a greater responsibility for the group agenda.

The key informants were impressed by the rapid success of the group program. They attributed this success to the fact that the program meets the needs of the seniors for social interaction and empowerment. They also credited the facilitators for the care and respect they show the elderly. One respondent especially commended the facilitators for encouraging seniors' comments and suggestions and for acting quickly on this feedback. Another key informant said that a focus on health issues in the group program and the administrative connection with a medical and dental clinic contributed to meeting urgent needs of the Vietnamese seniors.

RECENT DEVELOPMENTS

The group program is now offered on an ongoing basis. A lecture and discussion about electoral laws and customs was followed by elections where the Vietnamese older people chose representatives to sit on a Seniors' Committee. The members of this committee speak for those who are still reticent to make their desires known. The Seniors' Committee members also organize many celebratory events on their own and a few elders are learning to prepare and run the groups.

For a while, there was a monthly meeting of seven to ten older women about women's health issues, run by a Vietnamese trainee. The program was discontinued when the trainee left the center. However, the program was never very popular: Vietnamese women were not comfortable at being "segregated from the men," did not like the small group format, found it bothersome to come to the center twice a week, and were not impressed by the facilitator's skills.

Many subgroups of seniors now also meet regularly outside of the program. For example, a group of about ten women have started to meet at one another's houses once a week to socialize, and five

FIGURE 9.1

MULTICULTURAL FAMILY CENTER
Vietnamese Seniors Program

Goals: — Increase social interaction between Vietnamese seniors
              — Promote health and mental health
              — Empower Vietnamese older people
              — Foster integration to Canadian society

Format: — Drop-in
              — Every Tuesday from 11 a.m. to 4 p.m.
              — at Britannia Community Center (Seniors' Lounge)

Timeframe: 11:00 - 12:00   Body Checkup
              12:00 - 12:30   Gentle exercises
              12:30 - 1:00   Lunch (bring your own)
              1:00 - 2:30   Educational program/group discussion
              2:30 - 2:45   Break - refreshments
              2:45 - 4:00   ESL Clubs/Socializing/Practical help
                               (e.g., form filling)

Co-leaders: Lam Dang, cross-cultural facilitator
              Martine Levesque, social worker

SPRING - WINTER 1993 PROGRAM

Date	Body Checkup	Educational Program	Speaker
Jan 12	Introductory session		
Jan 19	Consultation Vancouver City Plan and Celebration Vietnamese New Year with children from Britannia Elementary		Stella Davis Social Planning Dpt - Vancouver
Jan 26	Workshop on depression and mental health (open to community)		Dr. Soma Ganesan VGH
Feb 2	Reflexology	Death #1	Group discussion
Feb 9	Medication REACH pharmacist	Death #2	Latinos French Canadians
Feb 16	Med consult. REACH doctor	Pet Therapy	BC Interact
Feb 23	Blood pressure REACH nurse	Safety	Chinatown Community Police
March 2	New foods REACH nutritionist	School system	Oakridge

Date	Body Checkup	Educational Program	Speaker
Mar 9	Foot care Vancouver General Hospital	Situation in Vietnam	University of British Columbia
Mar 16	Field trip to City Hall		
Mar 23	Dental screening REACH dentist and NHU hygienist	Home support services	North Health Unit (NHU)
Mar 30	Blood pressure REACH nurse	Housing	BC Housing
Apr 6	Field trip to Ukranian Center		
Apr 13	Medical consultation REACH doctor	Acupuncture	BC Acupuncture Society
Apr 20	Field trip to Citizenship Court		
Apr 27	Blood pressure REACH nurse	Respiratory diseases	Vancouver General Hospital
May 4	New foods REACH nutritionist	Customs regulations	Customs Canada
May 11	Field trip to Vancouver General Hospital		
May 18	Dental screening REACH dentist and NHU hygienist	Native issues	Native speaker
May 25	Last session. Socializing and evaluation.		

men regularly go swimming together. Other seniors organize their own community outings.

A subcommittee of seniors, assisted by the Vietnamese facilitator, successfully applied for a grant to produce pamphlets, radio programs, and a videorecording for Vietnamese seniors who do not know what services are available to them, or how to gain access to these resources. Meanwhile, some 30 Vietnamese elders have joined the ranks of a mainstream seniors' organization and are broadcasting monthly radio programs in Vietnamese on the social issues facing Vietnamese elderly.

The members of the group program have been consulted by the Social Planning Department of the City of Vancouver. They participated in an exhibition about their vision for Vancouver in the year 2000.

The group program now counts over 150 regular members (out of an estimated total of 600 Vietnamese seniors in Greater Vancouver), and membership is still increasing. A few group members volunteered that, although they are still economically dependent on their children, they have gained autonomy and their status within the family has increased in light of their knowledge of the community. Many of these older people, who two years ago may have been considered a burden on their family, have been instrumental in finding better and affordable housing, and are a source of information regarding legal, health, and resources issues for their community.

The success of the program is widely recognized. The Social Planning Department of the City of Vancouver is consulting the group program participants about permanent services for their cultural community, and the neighboring municipality of Surrey Delta started a similar support/education group program for its Vietnamese seniors.

It is interesting to note, following a lecture and discussion on family trees, a few group members stated that they would like to talk about the past. The majority, however, seemed uncomfortable with the emotionality of the topic. As the Vietnamese older people become more comfortable in the program, they may enjoy more intimate discussions. There is no pressure for this to happen, but care is taken not to hinder future developments by overprogramming or making decisions for the group members.

CONCLUSION

The experience of the group program with the Vietnamese older people reinforces the notion that flexibility, openness, and cultural sensitivity are the mainstays of social group work. In other words, by listening and responding, we were able to make changes that clearly made sense to the Vietnamese community and to the seniors in our group, who then encouraged more and more members to join them. Not only are these attributes necessary at the initial stage of a group program, but they are also indispensable both during planning and on an ongoing basis. In this case, the negative reaction of the Vietnamese Advisory Committee warned us of potential problems. We then modified the original program and prepared alternative approaches so that we could make changes on short notice. Later, continued attention to the feedback of the members permitted us to refine our interventions and, as participants became more comfortable and self-assured, they took more initiative inside and outside of the group program.

Both of the formal evaluations conducted credited much of the success of the group program to the care and the respect the facilitators showed the Vietnamese elders. This key factor is related to cultural sensitivity. In traditional Vietnamese culture, older people are worshipped and their authority within the family is undisputed (Dinh, Ganesan, and Waxler-Morrison, 1990). But older Vietnamese who move to Canada see their authority eroded by less respect for the elderly in Western cultures, loss of cultural and social competency, financial dependency on the family, and the need to learn English and adapt to Canadian life-styles. They are likely to be disheartened by their loss of public esteem and may feel that they have been betrayed. They are also extremely sensitive to signs of respect, especially from people perceived as "authorities." The two facilitators of the program made a point of treating the group members with the reverence they deserved and expected. They greeted the Vietnamese elders individually upon arrival and stood at the door to shake their extended hands before departure. They never interrupted people when they spoke, not even to ask them to be quiet at the beginning of a meeting. It would be impossible to mention all behaviors that conveyed their respect, but the most important point was that these behaviors were genuine, as both facilitators really enjoyed interacting with the members of the group.

Another critical sign of respect was that, from the very first session, the seniors really felt that the facilitators listened to their suggestions and feedback and that they acted quickly to make the desired changes to the program. A possible exception may be the still inadequate provision of child-care services, which is due to a tight budget. Any future expansion of the program will include child-minding services, which are particularly important for older

Vietnamese women, whose participation in the program declines significantly during school holidays.

Some factors of success are more difficult to identify because they are characterized by their absence rather than their presence. For example, this may be the case for religious and political neutrality. Respondents to the needs assessment survey (which preceded the implementation of the group program) stressed the importance of neutrality for those working with the Vietnamese, given the history of their home country which was divided into North and South Vietnam. There was much attention given to this factor during the planning of the group program and during debriefing sessions. We were vigilant to include everyone and are proud that group members are representative of all the religious and political affiliations present in the Vietnamese community.

The group experience made obvious what we know as group workers, but may not always take into account when working cross-culturally: what is appropriate for one cultural group is not necessarily appropriate for another. Group reminiscence may be an appropriate activity for Jewish immigrants, but the Vietnamese elders in Vancouver did not show much enthusiasm for it, mostly for cultural reasons, perhaps also because reminiscence was introduced too early in the life of the group. Group facilitators need to leave space for growth by providing opportunities for different types of exchanges and by not shunning emotional expression in its varied forms (Pearson, 1991).

The group program with Vietnamese older people has successfully tackled the four domains of multicultural social work with groups identified by Chau (1990): cultural adaptation, intragroup consciousness-raising and empowerment, intergroup relations, and ethnic rights. In 1986, Disman wrote, "Seniors are the most powerless, least influential, and most 'forgotten' segment of the ethnic population" (in Task Force, 1988, p. 79). The Multicultural Family Center's group program for Vietnamese elders represents an inexpensive, feasible, and exciting model to guard against this eventuality.

NOTE

1. Vietnamese informants stated that the low response rate was probably due to a combination of the following factors: many seniors cannot read or write, written

evaluations are most unusual in Vietnamese culture, and the evaluation form was crowded and difficult to read for those with bad eyesight. Moreover, the facilitators observed that spouses filled out only one evaluation form.

REFERENCES

Alcohol/Drug Education Service (1989). Alcohol/Drug Needs Assessment: Four British Columbia Ethnic Communities. Vancouver, BC.

Bernier, D. (1992). The Indochinese Refugee: A perspective from Various Stress Theories. *Journal of Multicultural Social Work, 2*,1: 15-29.

Breton, M. (1985). Reaching and Engaging People: Issues and Practice Principles. *Social Work with Groups, 8*, 3: 7-21.

Canadian Association of Schools of Social Work (1991). *Social Work Education at the Crossroads: The Challenge of Diversity.* Report of the Task Force on Multicultural and Multiracial Issues in Social Work Education. Ottawa: Canadian Association of Schools of Social Work.

Canadian Journal of Community Mental Health (1993). Special Issue of Cultural Diversity. *12*, 2.

Canadian Social Work Review (1991). Special issue on Multiculturalism and Social Work, *8.*

Canadian Task Force on Mental Health Issues Affecting Immigrants and Refugees (1988). *After the Door Has Been Opened.* Ottawa: Health and Welfare Canada.

Chau, K. (1990). Social Work with Groups in Multicultural Contexts. *Groupwork, 3*, 1: 9-21.

Chin, J. (1983). Diagnostic Considerations in Working with Asian Americans. *American Journal of Orthopsychiatry, 53*: 100-109.

Christensen, C. P. (1985). Perceived Problems and Help-Seeking Preferences of Chinese Immigrants in Montreal. *Canadian Journal of Counselling, 23*: 311-320.

Cox, C. (1982). Overcoming Access Problems in Ethnic Communities. In Gelfand, D. and C. M. Barresi (Eds.), *Ethnic Dimensions of Aging*, New York: Springer: 165-178.

Dinh, D.-K., S. Ganesan and N. Waxler-Morrison (1990). The Vietnamese. In Waxler-Morrison, N., J. Anderson and E. Richardson (Eds.) *Cross-Cultural Caring: A Handbook for Health Professionals in Western Canada.* Vancouver: University of British Columbia Press, Chapter 8: 181-213.

Disman, M. (1986). Aging and Ethnicity in Ontario. Toronto: not published.

Dorais, L.-J., L. Pilon-Le and H. Nguyen. (1987). *Exile in a Cold Land: A Vietnamese Community in Canada.* New Haven, CT: Yale Southeast Asia Studies.

Dowd, J. and V. Bengston (1978). Aging in Minority Populations: An Examination of the Double Jeopardy Hypothesis. *Journal of Gerontology, 33*: 427-436.

Fryer, M. (1992). Linking Schools of Social Work with Cultural Communities in Canada. Evaluation of the REACH Component: The Multicultural Family Center. Evaluation manuscript funded and submitted to Multiculturalism and Citizenship Canada. Unpublished.

Gardella, L. G. (1985). The Neighborhood Group: A Reminiscence Group for the Disoriented Old. Special issue on time as a factor in group work. *Social Work with Groups, 8*, 2: 43-52.

Gelfand, D. (1986). Assistance to the New Russian Elderly. *The Gerontologist, 26*: 444-448.

Glassman U. and L. Skolnik (1984). The Role of Social Group Work in Refugee Settlement. *Social Work with Groups, 7*, 1: 45-62.

Journal of Multicultural Social Work. (1992). Special Issue on Social Work with Immigrants and Refugees. 2.

Lee, J. (1987). Asian American Elderly: A Neglected Minority Group. In R. Dubrof (ed.), *Ethnicity and Gerontological Social Work.* Binghamton, NY: The Haworth Press, 103-116.

Lee, J., J. M. Patchner and P. Balgopal (1991). Essential Dimensions for Developing and Delivering Services for the Asian American Elderly. *Journal of Multicultural Social Work, 1*, 3: 3-11.

McNicoll, P. and C. P. Christensen (1993a). Direct Action: A School of Social Work Reaches Out to Cultural Communities. Unpublished paper.

_____ . (1993b). Linking School of Social Work with Cultural Communities: the Case of the Multicultural Family Center. Paper presented to the Learned Societies Conference in Ottawa, June 11, 1993.

Myerhoff, B. (1978). *Number Our Days.* New York: Simon and Schuster.

Pearson, V. (1991). Western Theory, Eastern Practice: Social Group Work in Hong Kong. *Social Work with Groups, 14*, 2: 45-58.

Ruthledge, P. J. (1992). *The Vietnamese Experience in America.* Bloomington and Indianapolis: Indiana University Press.

Tannenbaum, J. (1990). An English conversation group model for Vietnamese adolescent females. *Social Work with Groups, 6*, 2: 41-55.

Tribe, R. and J. Shackman (1989). A Way Forward: A Group for Refugee Women. *Groupwork, 2*: 159-166.

Tsui, P. and G. Schultz (1985). Failure of Rapport: Why Psychotherapeutic Engagement Fails in the Treatment of Asian Clients. *American Journal of Orthopsychiatry, 55*, 4: 561-569.

Wong, P. T. P. (1991). Social Support functions of group reminiscence. *Canadian Journal of Community Mental Health, 10*, 2: 151-161.

Chapter 10

Stages of Development in Women's Groups: A Relational Model

Linda Yael Schiller

INTRODUCTION

Groups move through distinct developmental stages as they progress through their life cycle, much as people do. It is important for the student of group work and the group facilitator to have a working understanding of the nature of this developmental course in order to better enhance the growth and change-producing components of the group for its members.

This chapter proposes that there is a different model of developmental stages for women's groups than for groups of men, mixed groups, or young children's groups. Drawing on the recent research into women's psychological development by feminist thinkers and the relational model they are proposing, as well as examining the different relationship women have with issues of power, status, and conflict, this chapter proposes that women's groups reflect these differences, and that normative group development for women follows a different course than it does for men. The facilitator who understands particular and unique patterns of growth and development can then intervene more effectively and in a style that best meets the differential needs of the group and its members at each stage of their development. A facilitator may choose a different intervention style for the same problem or dilemma depending on whether the group is in the early, middle, or final stages of its time together, and the facilitator's expectations regarding the development of her group may also affect its progress.

REVIEW OF THE "BOSTON MODEL" OF STAGES OF GROUP DEVELOPMENT

For many years one of the primary formulations for charting the developmental course of groups has been the five stages of what has become known as the "Boston Model." The ground-breaking work of Garland, Jones, and Kolodny (1978) set the tone for years to come, and has become a standard format in which group development has been described. Research cited in their article for the evolution of this conceptual framework is based primarily on the authors' experiences with facilitating groups of children and adolescents. They describe five stages of development for these groups: pre-affiliation; power and control; intimacy; differentiation; and separation. Each stage has its own dynamic themes, its own inherent issues and struggles, and its own implications for facilitator interventions.

Pre-affiliation is the time when members are trying to decide if this is really the group for them, with issues of trust and preliminary commitment at the foreground. Dynamic themes of approach-avoidance are common. The second stage of power and control is described as a universal time of status jockeying for positions of power and role within the group structure. It is seen as a time when members challenge the authority of the group facilitator, a time of testing limits and boundaries, and a time of competition and challenge amongst members. Once having sufficiently resolved this normative crisis, members are free to then move on to the third stage of intimacy, where connection and affiliation become more the norm, where risk-taking and self-disclosure are more evident, and interpersonal transferences become more pronounced. In this model, the fourth stage of differentiation is a time of greater self-expression and mutual support, a higher degree of group cohesion, and a more reality-based recognition of the individuals comprising the group (including the facilitator). Finally, the fifth stage of separation involves dealing with the impending loss of the group, with some inherent anxiety, regression and denial, recapitulation, review, evaluation, and letting go and separating.

VARIATIONS ON A THEME–
NORMATIVE DIFFERENCES

This chapter reexamines the application of the Boston model for a specific group population–the group comprised of and facilitated solely by women. It specifically examines the middle three stages, and proposes that for women's groups–those of adults and quite possibly older adolescent girls–there is a different yet normative developmental course. This different direction does not indicate unhealthy development. Nor does it imply that women's groups are skipping stages, and will then need to go back and recapitulate the earlier missed stage. Rather, it speaks to the fact that women's normative development, both within their life cycle in general and within groups, is different from that of men. This is an important distinction to make, for the new research on women's growth and development makes the point that normative developmental pathways seem different for girls than for boys. (Broverman et al. (1970) found a correspondence between what practitioners were defining as healthy adult functioning with characteristics they used to describe only men. They further discovered that practitioners identified characteristics describing some degree of mental illness or psychological impairment with characteristics they used to describe women.)

It is significant to recall that the existing model is based primarily on research and experiences with groups of young children, and that it was formulated by three scholarly men employing their own understandings and life experiences as males in groups in this society. Finally, the Boston model was originally formulated before the compilation of research based on feminist perspectives, and a growing recognition and understanding that there are significant differences in the way men and women define the importance and the place of relationships, power, and sense of self.

In recent years there has been an outpouring of new ideas about women's growth and development coming out of feminist inquiry into the nature of woman's experience. It is through this lens that the nature of women's experience in groups will also be examined.

FEMINIST THEORY, THE RELATIONAL MODEL, AND CONFLICT IN GROUPS

Starting with Miller (1976), theorists and practitioners have begun to understand the importance of relational development in framing a woman's sense of self in the world. She first noted the centrality of connection and affiliation for women, and how traditional theories of development from Freud through Erickson and others instead stress increasing independence and autonomy as the necessary hallmarks of growth and adult mental health. Subsequent work by Gilligan (1982) continues to explore the centrality of attachment and connection for a woman's sense of self, and how the importance of this basic experience of connectedness in the world profoundly influences a woman's ways of approaching conflict, disagreement, and confrontation.

Gilligan (1982), and later Stiver (1991) and Alonso (1992), speak of the difference in the way women define power, weaving it together with attention to attachment, relationship, and the care of others. This approach is in contrast to a model driven more by control, dominance, and status concerns. Tannen (1990) agrees that the main interactive "commodity" for men is hierarchy and status, while the main focus of concern and energy for women is intimacy. Tannen describes the difference between men's and women's ways of talking as the difference between "report-talk" and "rapport-talk." She describes the emphasis and intent for men in conversation as information sharing with attention to status and independence, while the emphasis and intent in conversation between women is seen as that of establishing affiliation, connection, and ofttimes mirroring or sameness.

Additionally, Tannen (1990) describes women's primary goals in conversation as a search for an expression of mutual understanding, a reinforcement of rapport by offering the message "I understand, you're not alone, I've felt like that too." Jordan (1991) refers to the clinical implications of what the Stone Center for Developmental Services and Studies at Wellesley College calls the relational model of women's development as a need to focus on and help facilitate the development of empathy and mutuality. In fact, "The Stone Center model suggests that . . . relationship, based on empathic attunement, is the key to the process of therapy, not just the backdrop" (p. 284).[1] Furthermore, Jordan continues, "Feeling connected and in contact with (others) often allows us our most profound sense of personal meaning and reality . . . " (pg. 289). It is through this framework, that of the centrality of connection and relationship in women's lives, and the difference in the dynamic of power for men and for women, that women's experience in groups will be examined.

One of the primary differences between groups with male members and those with only women is in the way that they deal with conflict. Perhaps because of the prime importance of connection and affiliation for women, they frequently tend to challenge or confront only after a sense of connectedness, personal identity within this connectedness, and safety have been established. Additionally, according to Miller (1976), conflict has traditionally been a taboo area for women.

Hartung Hagen (1983) discussed all-women groups and conflict. She acknowledges that while conflict is likely to occur in some capacity in most groups, "Most of the research on group development and member behaviors has been done in groups that included men." She hypothesizes that ". . . all-women groups may move through developmental stages . . . differently than groups with men members," and she also concurs that women's groups seem to work on issues involving intimacy earlier than groups with men. Finally, she too has observed that a fairly high degree of trust and safety must have occurred for members to feel comfortable allowing conflict to surface. From here, however, she diverges to discuss the socialization of women to avoid conflict, and techniques for conflict management in women's groups. Garvin and Reed (1983), in their discussion of gender issues in social group work, state that "Women and men are likely to use power and handle opportunities for intimacy differently from each other." The following model proposes that establishing connection and intimacy is a necessary prerequisite for the surfacing of conflict or the challenge of authority in women's groups.

This point is in contrast to the Boston model, which proposes that intragroup conflicts emerge more or less immediately following the pre-affiliation stage. The relational model proposed here stresses that members must first have established a sense of safety in their group affiliations and connections before they are able to take on and challenge each other. Furthermore, it is not at all clear that women's groups go through a power and control stage in the manner described in our existing research. The next section examines these concepts in greater detail.

WOMEN IN GROUPS–A RELATIONAL MODEL

The proposed model for women in groups is a five-stage model structured along the lines of the Boston model. It seems that the first and fifth stages are fairly universal: there is a preaffiliation time when members are assessing (internally or externally) the pros and cons of making the commitment to truly engage in the group process, and a time of separation and termination–of leave-taking, saying good-by, and moving on. However, the middle three stages seem different for women's groups.

This chapter is proposing that the middle three stages of development for women in groups are:

2. Establishing a relational base
3. Mutuality and interpersonal empathy
4. Challenge and change

The Second Stage: Establishing a Relational Base

Contrary to the prevailing mode of thinking, women's groups do not seem to move into a power and control stage after their initial preaffiliation. Instead, because of the centrality and importance of connection for women in their lives and in their healing process, they spend their time and energy in the second group stage establishing a common ground and a sense of connection with each other and with the facilitator. Women do not seem to feel the need to jockey for status and power at this juncture, if at all. Rather, this time is spent discovering similarities and common experiences, and seeking (sometimes anxiously) approval and connection from both the other group members and the facilitator. Establishing a relational base also seems to involve the establishment of a felt sense of safety within the group.

Women are so frequently disempowered in their lives that a sense of safety in the world at large or in a group is not something that is taken for granted. Safety must be established as a prerequisite to greater intimacy or self-disclosure. Evolving roles and status within the group during subsequent stages seem to emerge more from the content and quality of each woman's interactions with the other members, and from their perceptions of themselves and the others as possessing the capabilities for empathy, understanding, and support.

Three different group settings will illustrate this construct. While each of the three group settings described below are distinct from each other (adult survivors of sexual abuse, mothers connected with social services, and graduate social work students), it is important to acknowledge that to varying degrees these are all vulnerable populations. While it may be argued that all women's groups are groups involving a vulnerable population, it is important to remain sensitive to the possibility that the particular vulnerabilities of the populations used to illustrate may have had some influence on how the model itself was developed.

The first illustration of how this process develops was seen in a short-term (16-week) group for adult survivors of sexual abuse.

Because of the short-term nature of this group, as well as the amount of emotional investment the members make in a group of this type, it was expected that the preaffiliation stage would not last much past the first, or possibly second, session. During the second session, the members had this discussion.

Helene: You know, I was really anxious about joining this group. I was so afraid that this would be like the other groups I've been in before–I was too afraid to open my mouth in them. I always felt so different from everyone else.

Joanne: Me too. Different and judged–and not just when I've been in some kind of group–in lots of places in my life.

Carmen: You feel like you're starting out with some strikes against you right from the beginning. At least in this group I knew from the start that everyone would be a survivor. Even if you all haven't been through exactly the same thing I've been through, you've all been there in some way or another, or you wouldn't be in this group.

Facilitator: Whatever differences there may be between you, you all have a lot in common—you are all survivors of sexual abuse. That is one of the reasons that groups can be so power-ful—because, as Carmen said, you've all been there. You all have a lot to offer to one another and can really help each other in moving through this healing process.

Michele: This might sound really strange, but I've been really happy since last week. I've felt so "given to" by each of you, and good about myself that I was finally "giving myself" this group. It's also made me wonder whether my individual work-er has enough expertise, the way Linda and Bonnie (the facili-tators) do.

In this example, the reaching for connection, the desire to estab-lish sameness (or at least similarity) of experience and history, and with Michele, the bid for affection and approval from both the group members and the facilitators, are clearly observable. In He-lene's opening statement, she is reaching for connection as well as safety by indicating that she had not felt safe enough to speak up in other groups she had been in. In verbalizing her fears and anxieties at this juncture, she seems to be reaching for safety and assurances that this experience would be different. By the end of this meeting, many of the members had their shoes off, indicating their growing comfort with each other and the growing sense of safety that al-lowed them to let their guard down.

In the first two meetings, one member, Kathleen, had brought a teddy bear and a small blanket with her to the group. By the third meeting, several of the members were bringing stuffed animals or other comfort items, and Jo, who had not, asked Kathleen if she could borrow her bear to hold during the check-in.

The second illustration is a long-term open-ended mothers' group held at a local outpatient mental health clinic. Some of the mothers participating in the group had been flagged by the Department of Social Services as "at risk" mothers for abuse or neglect of their children. All of the mothers in the group struggled to balance the parenting of their children with the often harsh realities of their own lives, including poverty and other forms of oppression, single parenting, few support systems, a dysfunctional family of origin that offered no positive models for their own parenting, and no exposure to alternative styles of parenting.

Since this was an open-ended group, members were periodically added. Two new members, Donna and Karinne, joined the group after it had been meeting for almost a year. Because of the semi-mandated nature of the referrals (protective services often "suggested" that members participate, and at times made participation a formal part of their service plan), members frequently had a great deal of ambivalence about engaging. This stage of establishing a relational base would be crucial if members were to be able to get past feeling required to participate and become able to find within themselves the motivation and desire to attend. The group itself had already coalesced past this stage, and now needed to deal with the task of integrating the new members and helping them to "catch up" with the rest of the group. This is an excerpt from Donna and Karinne's fourth meeting.

> **Terry:** My kids were holy terrors this week. Jackie pulled that tantrum thing again and I thought that I would lose it.
>
> **Denise:** What was it about this time?
>
> **Terry:** Bedtime, what else. That seems to be her favorite time to throw a fit. I know we talked here about how everyone is tired by then, and that she's testing me, but that screaming really makes me crazy.
>
> **Denise:** Did you do that story thing, that bedtime thing with her that day?
>
> **Terry:** You know, now that you mention it, I didn't. We'd been out all day, and I was tired and just wanted her to go to bed.
>
> **Donna:** (this was her first time speaking since joining the group) What story thing?

Katie: Maybe we talked about it before you joined. It really helps. It's about having a bedtime ritual that's always the same to help the kids quiet down. Then they can count on it. Like we do here in group–we can count on it every week to have juice or coffee, to have the same rules every week, and that we'll all be here unless we're really sick or have an emergency.

Facilitator: That's right, Katie. When we know that we can count on each other to be consistent and respect the agreements that we have made with each other, then we grow to trust and count on each other here in the group. It works that way in families, too.

Donna: You mean, that if you do things the same way with kids so they can count on it, like a bedtime story, or the same punishment for the same crime, then they get better behaved?

Terry: Yeah, and I forgot about that the other day when my kid was having a fit. I went back to my old way of dealing with her, which never did work very well anyway.

Donna: Hmmm.

Facilitator: Do you have some thoughts or feelings about this, Donna?

Donna: Well, you know that I wasn't too crazy about the idea of joining this group in the beginning, but I have troubles handling my kids sometimes, too. They can take a fit and then I don't know what to do with them either. I love them, but sometimes they can be so hard.

Karinne: (also her first time speaking in the group since day one) Me, too. I don't want to hit them, but sometimes I can't think of nothing else to do.

Ellen: We're all like that–that's why we're here. But we get ideas and help from each other here. It's a good group.

In this second example, we see again the power and the importance of establishing the relational base before subsequent work can take place. The two new members in this open-ended group slowly allowed themselves to acknowledge the similarities between themselves and the other members, thus affirming their membership in the group by being "all in the same boat" (Shulman, 1992). As the, sense of connection and safety in the group became clearer, Karinne was able to make the not-so-veiled disclosure around her difficulties with appropriate discipline methods. As they ventured toward connection and affiliation with the longer-term members, they were met with inclusion and support, succinctly expressed by Ellen's words, "We're all like that, that's why we're here . . . "

In the third illustration, a classroom group setting (here looking at a social group work class composed solely of women), we still see the development of group stages that arise in more therapeutic groups. It is not unusual for students to enter the stage of establishing the relational base by the second or third class. This is when students began to make appointments to meet with the professor outside of class and to volunteer their past experiences in the classroom or in the field. In one class, when a student presented her anxiety about beginning to facilitate her first group, she was met by a resounding chorus of "Me too's" from her fellow students, who were relieved that someone had verbalized what they had been feeling. When an oral presentation in lieu of a final paper was an option, by the second and third class students were volunteering to present. Since at least one meeting with the professor was a requirement for the oral presentation, as well as providing accompanying written materials, it is not difficult to see the desire for connection being expressed, as well as the bid for approval, in this case from the facilitator/professor.

The Third Stage: Mutuality and Interpersonal Empathy

The third stage in women's groups corresponds with what Shulman (1992), and Schwartz (1971), call the work stage, and with what Germain and Gitterman (1980) call the ongoing phase. It also roughly corresponds with what Garland, Jones, and Kolodny (1978) call the intimacy stage. However, it seems to go beyond intimacy as it has been defined. This is the time when women's groups move past the establishment and recognition of their similarities and the connections that arise from them, and into a safe and sacred space of trust, disclosure, and recognition and respect for the differences among them, without sacrificing the connection in doing so. If the second stage of establishing the relational base has been successfully negotiated, women's groups next move on to a mutuality that allows room both for difference and for empathetic connection. This too is in contrast to the current Boston model, which postulates "intimacy" and "differentiation" as two separate stages.

The facilitator's role in all of these stages is crucial. If her basic philosophy is one that stresses mutuality both amongst members and between members and facilitators, and she believes in and promotes members helping members (a basic social group work philosophy which dovetails nicely with the philosophy of the Stone Center's work), then the group dynamics will be more likely to reflect her belief in the power of growth through connection. Klein (1972) stresses that the facilitator operates from a stance or position vis-à-vis the healing process of the group, and that a clear, comfortable, and syntonic philosophy around this operating stance helps the members to achieve their goals in the group. Surrey (1991) suggests that "[Facilitators] direct their attention to the relational context. . . ." Jordan (1991) suggests that this empathic attunement is marked by intimacy and mutual intersubjectivity, defined as ". . . an interest in, attunement to, and responsiveness to the subjective inner experience of the other at both a cognitive and affective level." Furthermore,

> While some mutual empathy involves an acknowledgment of sameness in the other, an appreciation of the differentness of the other's experience is also vital. The movement toward the other's differentness is actually central to growth in relationships and also can provide a powerful sense of validation for both self and others.[2]

A powerful example of the transition to the third stage of mutuality and interpersonal empathy occurred in a social group work class. The class was discussing implications of oppression in their work in the fourth or fifth class of the semester, and had been asked by the professor to reflect on the first time that they had experienced a sense of oppression in their own lives. The professor shared her first experience with oppression in the form of anti-Semitism while in junior high school. Since it was almost the end of the class period, the students were asked to reflect on this over the week, and to share their experiences or memories next week. The following week the professor opened the class with the invitation to share experiences they may have recalled. The hand of an African-American student, Anna, shot up immediately. She said:

> I thought of something almost right away that I hadn't thought about in years, and hadn't really thought about as oppression before. I just knew that it made me feel so angry and left such a bad taste in my mouth. When I was about five years old, I spent the summer on a sort of camp/farm with a white family. My mother had carefully prepared my hair with the braids and the oil in our tradition to make it look really special, since I was going away. The very next day after I arrived at the place, the woman took me into the bathroom for my bath and said something like, "Now we'll get you looking all pretty for company tonight," and proceeded to undo all my braids and wash the oil out of my hair. She didn't know a thing about black hair! I remember feeling so humiliated and so mad for all the work my mother had put into it. I was only five years old though, and didn't know how to explain to her what she was doing to me, sort of washing away my pride.

There was a moment in the room when one could feel the energy shift to a deeper level. Then other class members, predominantly Caucasian, responded with expressions of empathy, of outrage at the insensitivity of the woman, and of true and heartfelt appreciation to Anna for sharing her poignant tale. A fruitful and thoughtful discussion took place in which other class members risked some personal self-disclosure following Anna's lead. In spite of the fact that no two stories were the same, and that women of color were a distinct minority in this classroom, a sense of safety in risk-taking had been established, and the very expression of their differences forged a bond among them. It was truly the moment in this classroom group when a shared and sacred space was created, interpersonal empathy was expressed and felt, and differences were acknowledged and respected within the larger context of connection, all hallmarks of this developmental stage.

The Fourth Stage: Challenge and Change

It seems to be a truth that for growth to occur, one must confront and challenge old or outdated ideas about oneself, one's way of relating in the world, and/or one's interpersonal relationships. In groups, sometimes this growth occurs through one's own emerging awareness, though often it occurs as someone else challenges or confronts a cherished thought or perception. The intricate dynamics between power and authority on one hand, and conflict, relatedness, and connection on the other, often emerge in a group of women during this fourth stage much as a cleansing, releasing wind. During this stage, if women have sufficiently experienced connection, empathic attunement, and respect for differences, they are now free to challenge themselves, each other, and the facilitators.

When the premise for this chapter was mentioned in an all-women social group work class, one of the members of this classroom group responded, "Oh, I agree. I couldn't imagine disagreeing with someone in a group until I was sure that they liked me first!" Imbedded in what this student said about not being able to confront unless she was sure that she was liked first, is the implication that if she did feel "liked" (that is, that she experienced a sense of empathic connected respect from the other members and from the facilitator), she would then be able to constructively challenge or confront without fear of losing her place or her sense of self in the process.

The traditional Boston model calls the time of "negotiating the problems of status, ranking, communication and influence" and "the time of dealing with issues of rebellion and testing authority" the power and control stage, following preaffiliation, and resulting in a hierarchical status arrangement within the group. As previously discussed, women have a different set of needs following their initial decision to engage in the group which involves the establishment of safety and connectedness; but they do not seem to be as concerned or involved with the issues of status or ranking at any point in the group cycle. Tannen (1990) describes a study by Johnstone involving community and contest that concludes that men see power as coming from an individual acting in opposition to others and to natural forces, and that life is seen as a contest. This fits with our understanding of the power and control stage for men. She goes on to conclude that for women, community is the source of power, and that for women the danger is being cut off from the community.

Miller (1976) states that "women do not need to set affiliation and strength in opposition to each other," and that "women do not have a history of believing that their power is necessary for maintenance of self-image." She goes on to describe power for women today as "the capacity to implement," making the distinction between "power for oneself" and "power over others," a distinction that might also be viewed as the difference between "power with" and "power over." In a later work, Miller (1991) describes women's experiences with use of their power in the world (that is, experiences with challenging or confronting others or expressing for oneself an unpopular or contradictory viewpoint). What she calls "the troublesome equations" include women's experiences of equating power with selfishness, destructiveness, and/or abandonment. That is, if a woman uses her power, she may precipitate attack and thus abandonment, which threatens a central part of her identity based on connectedness.

Given a history of women's general disempowerment, the experience of power as a taboo subject, and the "troublesome equations" with power, this important stage in group development can be the time when women take some real leaps of faith, and experiment on the cutting edge of their own growth. The challenge of this stage of growth is to maintain and even enhance the connections they have been forging. Simultaneously, they allow themselves to question authority, to challenge themselves and each other, and to risk the direct expressions of anger, disappointment, dissatisfaction, and disagreement without fear of losing the valuable threads of connection. The following two examples illustrate how this "challenge" effects change.

In the first example, a short-term group for adult survivors of sexual abuse followed a model that included a week for each woman to tell her story, to share with the group her history of abusive experiences as well as anything else she wanted to share about her life, her history, and her healing process. This part of the group experience was clarified for each woman during the initial screening interview. About two-thirds of the way through the group cycle, all but two women had taken their turn. One of the two remaining women, Lisa, had become increasingly quiet and withdrawn during the past few weeks. She initially had been engaged and participatory, but had lately described feeling shut off from the others, and in her own world. She spoke of her "turtle shell" retreat, a place familiar to her in her world outside of the group as well. The other group members and the facilitators had responded to her both with respect for her needs and pacing, as well as with attempts to keep her engaged and connected.

One week Lisa stayed after the group to tell the facilitators that she did not think she would be able to take her turn at telling her story as he other members had. She spoke of how difficult it was for her to share anything. The facilitators pointed out how her ability to make that statement was in essence her way of sharing and connecting at this point in time, and encouraged her to both be true to herself and her own needs for safety and to simultaneously consider if there were ways that she might be able to take her turn while honoring that need. Additionally, the facilitators pointed out that the decision as to how she would participate was ultimately hers to make, but that it was "group business" and could not remain a "secret" discussion, and thus needed to be brought up at the following group meeting.

The following week, Lisa announced to the group that she did not think she could share her story with the group. The facilitators noticed a wave of silent reaction spread through the group when Lisa made her announcement, and asked Lisa if she would be willing to hear feedback and reactions from the group regarding her decision. When Lisa indicated that she was willing to hear reactions, the other members responded.

> **Diana:** You know, Lisa, I feel really angry with you for disappearing on us here. We all came here for the same reason, and it feels unfair that you aren't willing to take the same risks that we do.

> **Ruth:** We've talked about how this was the reason we joined a group at all–so we could support and share with each other what we've been through. I guess I'll feel angry, too, if you don't take your turn.

Marissa: I'll feel disappointed. I really looked forward to hearing from you when you spoke before. I'll miss it if you don't now.

Lisa: Well, I guess I can't blame you if you're angry with me. I'd probably be angry with me, too.

Jes: You know, I wonder what you're thinking when you sit there and don't talk. I worry that you're judging the rest of us or something.

Lisa: Judging? Not at all. It never occurred to me that you could be thinking that! Do you others think that, too?

Diana: Well, it has crossed my mind. I know that this is hard stuff–it's hard for all of us–but I haven't been able to figure out what happened to make you so silent after the first few weeks.

Lisa: It wasn't anything that you (indicating the group as a whole) did. Wow, I had no idea that just my not talking would have any effect on other people. I guess I have a lot to think about–this certainly isn't the first time this has happened to me.

Facilitator: Do you have any second thoughts, Lisa, about taking a turn for your story?

Lisa: Well, I guess I'll go next week–but I can't promise anything detailed.

Facilitator: I don't think anyone is asking you to, Lisa. It seems more like the group–including us (referring to the facilitators)–cares about you, and misses your feedback.

This vignette illustrates the power of women finding their voice, and directly challenging and confronting a member about her behavior. (The facilitator here is facing the struggle around how to be with both the group and the individual. The work may have become split when Lisa stayed after group to speak with the facilitators alone the previous week.) Earlier on in the group, the members had held back on expressing their growing feelings of anger, resentment, and disappointment in order to pay attention to the tasks of connecting, affiliating, and forming a safe atmosphere of mutuality and empathy. These tasks accomplished, they could now challenge not only Lisa, but also themselves to express directly what they had been feeling without fears of abandonment or retribution from the group. Lisa herself was able to listen without becoming defensive, perhaps because she could hear the caring imbedded in their message to her. What Shulman (1992) calls the "demand for work" in a group, here expressed as a challenge for growth, was taken by Lisa, as she not only agreed to tell her story, but indicated that the group's challenge had led her to some important introspection about how she appeared to others outside of the group as well.

The second example of this stage is a mothers' group for women whose children had been sexually abused. The women had been meeting for about three-quarters of a year. Up until this point in time, the prevailing mood of the group in relation to the perpetrators had been one of anger, some revenge fantasies, and some confusion. It had been the established "norm" in the group not to express any affection for the perpetrator, nor a desire to maintain contact with him, aside from lamenting the financial losses. The issue of possible conflicting loyalties had remained just under the surface, while on the face of things, the women were "100 percent" behind their children. Jody missed a meeting one week, and the following week the members checked in to find out why.

> **Candace:** How come you didn't come to group last week, Jody?
>
> **Jody:** Well, I had an appointment. (A short silence) Actually, had to go to the prison to visit Bill.
>
> **Tina:** You what? Why did you have to go? That scum.
>
> **Jody:** Well, I had to talk to him about some things.
>
> **Debbie:** Why couldn't your social worker just give him a message for you?
>
> **Jody:** (Taking a deep breath) Well, I kind of wanted to talk to him in person. Myself.
>
> **Tina:** What on earth for?
>
> **Jody:** Well, even though he did some bad things to the kids, I still think about him sometimes. He wasn't all bad, you know. And I just needed to see how he was–jail can be pretty rough.

Tina: I can't believe you said that. I hate my "ex"–if I never see him again it would be too soon.

Jody: Well, everyone's different. You know, before I found out what he was accused to doing to the kids, I thought he was pretty good. He never beat me or anything, like your "ex" did. (Turning to facilitators) What do you think?

Facilitators: Does anyone else have something to add first? (The other members decline and look to facilitators) This is a pretty tricky issue for everyone, and Jody's certainly right that "everyone's different." It took a lot of courage for Jody to bring this up today, since I'm pretty sure that she knew that not everyone would agree with her. As a matter of fact, it seems to push some real buttons for some of you. As hard as it might have been for Jody to say, it might have been equally as hard for some of you to hear.

Jody: You're not kidding. I wasn't sure I was going to mention it, but then I decided, "What the heck," if I can't say it here, where can I talk about it?

Leslie: Yeah, I don't even like to talk about it. But, it's O.K. that you said it, Jody. I mean, it's not for me, but like you said, everyone's different.

Facilitator: It seems like what Jody is saying to us, is that she trusted the group enough to say something that she was pretty sure people might not agree with. So whether people agree with her wanting to see Bill or not, it seems like she made us a gift by telling us about her feelings. It really shows how far we've all come as a group, that there's enough trust to risk saying scary things.

Tina: I know that there's no love lost for me, but I can see where your situation might be different.

Jody: Well, thanks.

In this second vignette, we see a member take on, or challenge an unspoken rule in the group, that of "don't talk about any loyalty conflicts or positive feelings about the offender." Although understandably hesitant to bring it up, she took the risk at this stage of the group's development, trusting enough in her own strength to potentially disagree, and in the group's strength to both accommodate difference and maintain connection. This is a variation on the first example, where the group was challenging an individual member. Here, we see a member challenge a group norm.

The role of the facilitator again is critical. The challenge for the facilitator, perhaps especially at this stage, is to support both the individual and the group at the same time, and to help provide a climate in which "challenge and change" can safely unfold. The facilitator works to acknowledge with the group that conflict and connection are able to exist simultaneously.

CONCLUSION

From the above discussion, a critical examination of the notion that stages of development are the same for groups that include men and for groups that are composed of solely women can begin. Women's different ways of relating in groups have been discussed, and primary differences in the value and importance women and men place on power, status, and relational connections have been cited as some of the factors which influence the different developmental path women's groups follow.

This chapter proposes that women's developmental path in a group is composed of these five stages: pre-affiliation; establishing a relational base; mutuality and interpersonal empathy; challenge and change; and separation and termination. While the first and last stages have been viewed as fairly consistent with other groups, the middle three stages have been explored as unique to women's groups by examining them both through the perspective of social group work theory and the perspective of feminist inquiry.

Implications for future research and practice include exploring the relationship and connection between a facilitator's philosophical stance and her expectations from her group, and the way in which the group actually evolves. For the facilitator who espouses this relational model, some of the goals for her facilitation would be a nonhierarchical model, one which enhances and encourages connection and recognizes the power and primacy of relationships for growth and healing. She would also recognize the importance of a felt sense of safety within the relationships before she would encourage members to challenge themselves, each other, or the authority figure. Hopefully, if a nonhierarchical model were put into practice, the differential between the power and authority of the facilitator and the group members would be at a minimum, and members would feel empowered, rather than intimidated, by opportunities that arose for this cutting-edge growth in the group.

Finally, additional research on women's groups and their stages of development would be useful for enhancing our knowledge and, thus, our practice with this powerful mode of growth and healing of women in groups.

NOTES

1. It can be noted here that the therapeutic relationship and an empathic attunement is of critical importance for both men and women. It may be, however, that the timing of the attention to the relationship may have greater primacy to women.

2. We know that groups and their development can be powerfully influenced by their facilitators' basic style and by their interventions in the group. An interesting question might be whether men's or children's groups would follow similar paths if the facilitation were skillful. In a similar vein, do power struggles or a separation of intimacy and differentiation occur because we expect them to, or because they are inherently normative?

REFERENCES

Alonso, A. (1992). "Women's Development and Group Psychotherapy: A Fortuitous Synergy," in *Developments*, 1:1, p. 5.

Broverman, I. K., Broverman, D. M., Clarkson, R. E., Rosencrantz, P. S., and Vogel, S. R. (1970). "Sex Role Sterotypes and Clinical Judgments of Mental Health," in *Journal of Consulting and Clinical Psychology*, 34, No. 1, 1-7.

Garland, J.; Jones, H.; and Kolodny, R. (1978). "A Model for Stages of Development in Social Work Groups," in S. Bernstein, ed., *Explorations in Group Work*, Boston, MA: Charles River Books, 17-71.

Garvin, C. D. and Reed, B. G. (1983). "Gender Issues in Social Group Work: An Overview," in *Social Work with Groups*, 6:3/4, 5-18.

Germain, C. B. and Gitterman, A. (1980). *The Life Model of Social Work Practice*, New York: Columbia University Press.

Gilligan, C. (1982). *In a Different Voice*, Cambridge, MA: Harvard University Press.

Hartung Hagen, B. (1983). "Managing Conflict in All-Women Groups," in *Social Work with Groups*, 6:3/4, 95-104.

Jordan, J. (1991). "Empathy, Mutuality and Therapeutic Change: Clinical Implications of a Relational Model," in Jordan, J. V., Kaplan, A. G., Miller, J. B., Stiver, I. P., and Surrey, J. L. *Women's Growth in Connection, Writings from the Stone Center*, New York: The Guilford Press, 283-290.

Klein, A. F. (1972). *Effective Groupwork*, New York: Association Press.

Miller, J. B. (1976). *Toward a New Psychology of Women*, Boston: Beacon Press.

_____ . (1991). "Women and Power," in *Women's Growth in Connection, Writings from the Stone Center*, New York: The Guilford Press, 197-205.

Schwartz, W. (1971). "On the Use of Groups in Social Work Practice," in W. Schwartz and S. Zalba, eds., *The Practice of Group Work*, New York: Columbia University Press, 3-24.

Shulman, L. (1992). *The Skills of Helping Individuals and Groups*, Itasca, IL: F. E. Peacock Publishers, Inc.

Stiver, I. P. (1991). "The Meaning of Care: Reframing Treatment Models," in Jordan, J. V., Kaplan, A. G., Miller, J. B., Stiver, I. P., and Surrey, J. L. *Women's Growth in Connection, Writings from the Stone Center*, New York: The Guilford Press 250-267.

Surrey, J. L. (1991). "Relationship and Empowerment," in Jordan, J. V., Kaplan, A. G., Miller, J. B.,Stiver, I. P., and Surrey, J. L. *Women's Growth in Connection, Writings from the Stone Center*, New York: The Guilford Press, 112-180.

Tannen, D. (1990). *You Just Don't Understand: Women and Men in Conversation.* New York: Morrow.

Chapter 11

Adversity, Diversity, and Empowerment: Feminist Group Work with Women in Poverty

Anna Travers

This chapter describes the evolving work of a small, grass roots women's organization, Opportunity for Advancement, in Toronto, Canada. For almost 20 years, the agency has been offering groups for women living on welfare who want to make changes in their lives–changes that promise a pathway out of grinding poverty, or that break down isolation and despair, or that offer some control over experiences of trauma and victimization.

Although not publicly described as "feminist" in the beginning, the model that was developed was clearly based in feminist values such as choice, the validation of personal experience, a recognition of women's work both in and outside the home (and the tensions between the two), and the need to confront societal barriers faced by women, especially single mothers (Browne, Filger, and McDonald, 1989).

More recently, there has been a recognition in the women's movement that we must look at all forms of oppression in an integrated way, particularly the effects of racism and classism as they interact with sexism (Weir, 1987; Fulani, 1987). At Opportunity for Advancement, this has been reflected in a continued emphasis on the interplay between gender and economic relations, as well as an increased commitment to working explicitly with women on the impact of racism in their lives, and to increasing the diversity of our organization. Other forms of discrimination based on categories such as age, marital status, ability, or sexual orientation are likewise named and challenged. An effort is made to balance the struggle against prejudice by learning about and affirming racial, cultural, and social differences.

This chapter will describe the group work model, "Preparing for Change," that is used to empower women facing multiple oppressions. First, it will briefly outline the way in which recent Canadian social policy reflects public attitudes about women, especially single mothers, so as to provide the economic and ideological context for our work. Then, it will describe the women we serve and their life situations, and explain how feminism provides the theoretical framework on which our understanding and values are based. Lastly, it will discuss the purpose of the group and illustrate how our practice is informed by this feminist perspective as well as other approaches such as social group work and popular education.

AN OVERVIEW OF SOCIAL PROGRAMS FOR SINGLE MOTHERS IN CANADA

Social policies toward single mothers in Canada have always been a barometer by which to measure attitudes about families, the division of roles and responsibilities between men and women, and concepts of "worthiness." In Ontario, for example, widows were first given financial benefits in 1920, while other single mothers–women who had never married or were divorced–had to wait until the mid-1950s to become eligible (Evans, 1991).

Throughout the past 60 years in Canada, and in most Western societies, women have been subjected to contradictory demands and ambiguous messages. There has been a continuing tension between the work ethic and the family ethic, between the demands of production and reproduction, which the government has tried to mediate through various social policies and incentives. During the 1950s and 1960s, there was an entrenchment of the ideology of separate functions within the family structure in the form of familial patriarchy–man as breadwinner and woman as homemaker–buttressed by generous state support of the family and restrictions on women's access to the paid labor force (Ursel, 1992). Single mothers raising children were entitled to long-term state support, albeit at subsistence levels, because, like women in two-parent families, they were fulfilling sex-role expectations.

By the 1970s, these social arrangements were starting to break down as the development of multinational corporations and the use of a global labor force with cheaper labor costs made the "family wage" untenable. In the last 15 years, there has been a movement of women into the work force in unprecedented numbers. In 1989, 67 percent of mothers with children under 16 were employed, the majority full-time (Statistics Canada, 1992). In addition to wanting a wider range of occupational choices than just homemaking, women have been forced to work outside the home in order to maintain an adequate standard of living. Single-parent mothers, however, even when employed, are particularly vulnerable to poverty because, as Evans (1990) points out, "the barriers to adequate earnings—low pay and occupational segregation that confront all women in the labor market—make it extremely difficult for single mothers to earn an income that brings the household above the poverty line" (1990, p. 182).

Presently, we are seeing increasing economic continentalization (NAFTA, the EEC) and a concomitant dismantling of the welfare state, exemplified in Canada by policies such as the reduction of federal transfer payments, cutbacks in child-care subsidies, and deinstitutionalization. Ursel (1992) explains it thus:

> A dilution of the powers of the nation state seems essential to continental economic strategies. On the other hand, history indicates that the development and operation of a welfare state is premised on a centralization of powers at a federal level. As the two processes proceed in opposite directions, we understand that the global pursuit of lower waged labor and the continental organization of production is the latest strategy for capital's flight from the costs of reproducing labor. (p. 303)

As public expenditures for services for children and the elderly are cut back and as subsidies for transportation and housing decline, the impact on women is far greater than on men. Women are not only the main recipients but also the providers of these services and are, therefore, losing out on both ends. Yet, as Armstrong and Armstrong (1987) points out,

> fewer and fewer women can rely on male financial support, and as more and more of them seek paid employment, they have less time, fewer resources, and often little desire to provide at home or in the volunteer sector what the state fails to provide in the public sector. Indeed, many of the services the state is threatening to "deinstitutionalize" and place in unpaid women's hands have never been in the home. (pp. 220-21)

Single mothers, now as ever, seem to be caught in the cross-fire between the countervailing pressures at work in Canada today. Current Ontario government proposals for welfare reform reflect the increasing expectation that all able-bodied women enter the work-force (Government of Ontario, 1988, 1993), but there are neither the training programs, the child-care services, nor the jobs to make such an expectation feasible.

Opportunity for Advancement provides programs for women in this conflicting environment. Funded by provincial and municipal levels of government, the agency has a mandate to provide preemployment group programs for women on social assistance. Indeed, most of the women who participate are eager to leave social assistance provided they can earn sufficient wages. And yet, for all the reasons outlined above, the situation for women without job skills or experience, especially immigrants, older women, and those with children, is growing more difficult.

For group workers, torn between the women's needs, government mandates, and social realities, the frustrations are intense. It is vital to develop a clear analysis of economic and social conditions, so that we blame neither our participants for being "unmotivated" nor ourselves for being "incompetent," and so that we can share this analysis with the women themselves. It is also essential that the goals of the program, while supporting women who are trying to become economically self-sufficient, allow for a broader range of outcomes that enable women to improve the quality of their lives in other ways (e.g., decreasing isolation and participating in their communities; gaining access to appropriate housing, health care, or legal services; or using the emotional and practical support to rebuild lives shattered by abuse). At a broader level, the agency attempts to address gaps in services and contradictions in policy by participating in several coalitions and task forces, and offering education and training workshops on women and poverty.

WOMEN IN POVERTY: A FEMINIST UNDERSTANDING

Each year, Opportunity for Advancement runs 16 "Preparing for Change" groups in four inner-city neighborhoods in Toronto. This program serves over 225 women living on social assistance (General Welfare or Family Benefits), most of them caring for dependent children. Severe poverty is a given, as these women and children belong to a group that is more likely to be poor than any other in Canada. A 1991 report found that, on average, single parent mothers with children under 18 were living on annual incomes that were $9,051 below the poverty line (National Council of Welfare, 1993). In a large city like Toronto, it is impossible for a family on welfare to pay for adequate housing *and* cover basic food costs unless they are living in subsidized housing. As a result, overcrowded and dangerous apartments together with hunger or inadequate nutrition are facts of life. A 1989 study showed that 65 percent of the families using the Daily Bread downtown food bank in Toronto were headed by single parents even though they represented only 15 percent of all families (referred to in Evans, 1991).

Agency statistics for 1993 show that about two-thirds of group participants were born in countries other than Canada and about half are women of color. The racial and cultural mix in the groups reflects the reality of Toronto as a magnet for immigrants and refugees from all over the world, as well as the work of the agency in reaching out to these populations. In the past few years, newcomers from Western Europe, the Caribbean, and South and Central America have been joined by new waves of immigrants and refugees from Eastern Europe, the Middle East, and Africa. Immigrant women on welfare face all the same issues as Canadian-born women, as well as a shortage of English language classes (especially ones with built-in child care), the need for settlement services and, frequently, systemic racism. Refugees may have difficulties related to their unchosen status as exiles from their own countries and to traumatic experiences suffered before they left. In addition, under Canadian law, most refugee claimants are not allowed to work and have to accept welfare until their hearings, a process which may take years.

Diversity is represented not only in terms of race and culture, but across almost every social category. In terms of age, the range is from 20 to over 60, although the majority (70 percent) of women are between 25 and 45. Older women without much education or previous attachment to the paid labor force find it even harder to get jobs, especially since training programs geared to their specific needs are being phased out. Considerable variety is also seen in educational levels: just over half the group members have less than a 12th grade education; some are barely literate; and a sizeable number (48 percent) have high school diplomas or some post-secondary education. It is usually the immigrant women who have higher levels of education, and who may also have held skilled jobs in their own countries, but their credentials and experience are often unrecognized in Canada.

Many, perhaps the majority, of the women have experienced violence or trauma in their childhood or adult lives. Most now live alone, in sole charge of dependent children, and often separated from networks of family or friends who could provide material and emotional support. Loneliness, exhaustion, and the emotional vulnerability that results from abuse are commonplace, and are exacerbated by poverty and social stigma (Dhillon and Walter, 1993). The lack of appropriate, accessible counselling services means that problems often build to crisis proportions. Many women end up as psychiatric patients, not because they seek this treatment, but because they have no other recourse. Labelling, drugging, and institutionalization do little to heal the psychic wounds–and may well add new ones (Lepischak, 1992).

The issues that the women bring to the groups–poverty, social isolation, lack of education, poor housing, physical and sexual abuse, discrimination, health problems, children who are failing at school, lack of access to services, dependency on prescription or street drugs, depression, and hopelessness–although disturbing and overwhelming, are probably familiar to the majority of workers in urban social agencies. What may be different in a feminist organization is the frame of reference that is used to understand these issues and, by extension, the goals and methods that are chosen to deal with them.

Mainstream social work, in which various theories and methods are integrated under the paradigm of systems theory, acknowledges that problems stem from difficulties between the individual and society. The systems perspective, or unitary approach, views society as a generally functional, organic entity consisting of interdependent units (Pincus and Minahan, 1973; Goldstein, 1973). This theoretical stance, together with the casework method that is the usual mode of intervention in social work, means that efforts are directed primarily at helping individuals and families adjust or develop better coping skills within existing social conditions (Carniol, 1987). It is a short step then, given this orientation and the pervasive influence of the medical model in social work, to defining problems themselves in terms of individual deficits or family dysfunction.

Critics of the systems or unitary perspective (Lewis, 1992; Langan, 1985) point out that it has an inherently conservative bias and that it avoids dealing with relationships based on exploitation. Langan argues that "the historical concepts of the unitary approach and its presumption of accepted moral values and social harmony obscure social conflict while upholding existing power relations" (p. 35). She believes that this has been particularly detrimental to women who constitute the majority of social work clients.

Other theorists (Loewenstein, 1976; McNay, 1992), while aware of the shortcomings of systems theory, still see its value in highlighting the interactions between social systems and in locating avenues for intervention. They propose the addition of an overall framework based on an analysis of power relations (particularly those derived from gender, class, and race perspectives) to provide a clarification of the values and goals of social work intervention. The role of the worker then is directed to helping clients to articulate their needs and understand the social forces that block the realization of these needs. Intervention involves the mutual development of techniques and strategies to address these barriers at whatever level (micro or macro) seems appropriate. This model would describe the feminist theoretical framework that currently underpins group work, individual counselling, and social action at Opportunity for Advancement.

In the field of social group work, as in social work in general, there has been a failure to acknowledge the fundamental lack of control, dependence, and alienation experienced by oppressed people. Breton (1992) argues that group work models such as the "social action" and "reciprocal" models, with their assumptions of responsible citizen participation on the one hand, and symbiotic interdependence between the individual and society on the other, are inappropriate and even victim-blaming when applied to disenfranchised people such as the homeless, the very poor, and those facing multiple oppressions. Breton calls for a "political action" model in the spirit of the "conscientization" movement practiced in Latin America, but sees the major stumbling block as the reluctance on the part of social workers to "let go of some of our power as professionals and experts" (Breton, 1992, p. 265).

Lee (1992), drawing on the antioppression pedagogy of Freire, also calls for a redefinition of role and purpose in social group work:

> Let us help group members to work on the complex person-environment transactions in the economic, social and political context in which they exist. Let us learn to trust the group, and to believe in people, to know that through the process of dialogue and mutual aid, we can find a way to do what needs to be done. It is not ours to know answers or teach or manipulate, or to lead in reform or revolution. It is ours to provide opportunities for people to come together in dialogic communication. (p. 19)

Since the goal of feminist social work is empowerment, even as the group tackles the complex task of deconstructing the attitudes, terms of language, institutions, and social structures by which inferior status is maintained, it must remain accessible to the participants and responsive to their priorities. Feminist practice avoids needless abstraction and reduces power differences between the worker and the participants by using everyday language rather than psychological jargon, by grounding analysis in concrete experience (women telling their own stories), and by rejecting the primacy of the worker as the one who defines (or worse, diagnoses) the problem and hence specifies the solution. The shifts from theory to practice, analysis to action, are seamless and dialectical as Levine (1982) describes:

> . . . there is a rejection of the artificial split between internal feelings and external conditions of living and working, between human behavior and structural context. A feminist approach to working with women involves weaving together personal and political issues as causes of and potential solutions to women's struggles. Women's struggles are placed within, not outside their structural context. (p. 200)

Feminist principles have been applied in various types of group work such as consciousness raising, mutual aid, political organizing, and healing work. The model developed at Opportunity for Advancement combines several of these features in a structured support group that offers women a place to share their problems, discover their strengths, develop new understandings of the social and political forces at work in their lives, and make plans for individual and collective action. Structure gives the program a coherence and intensity that would otherwise be hard to achieve given the diversity of the participants and the range of issues that the women bring to the groups. While the model was not consciously based on Popular Education principles, there are striking resonances between the two which will be highlighted in the next section.

"PREPARING FOR CHANGE": A GROUP FOR WOMEN IN POVERTY

Women on welfare are often described by social service providers as "unmotivated" or "hard to reach." In fact, it is often the services themselves that are hard to reach; and the manner in which they are delivered frequently reinforces the disempowered status of the recipient. Feminist services attempt to be accessible and to offer clients dignity by attending to the barriers that prevent poor and marginalized women from participating in programs, and by communicating autonomy and choice from the outset.

At Opportunity for Advancement, material supports such as on-site child care, bus tickets, and food are provided, and groups are located in familiar surroundings such as housing projects, community centers, and churches, close to public transportation. It is recognized that many potential participants, especially visible minority and immigrant women, are not connected with other services and may be totally isolated in their homes. In order to reach these women directly, a pair of outreach workers (usually former participants) distribute flyers, set up information tables in shopping malls, and knock on doors in public housing. Self-referrals are welcomed, information and encouragement are given, and the women themselves decide whether the program will meet their needs.

Strategies that make the programs accessible and inclusive also create increased challenges for both group members and the group worker. Neither the size nor the composition of the group is predictable at the outset, and the worker begins each new group wondering whether seven or 17 women will come, and whether there will be enough common ground for the women to bond with each other. The diversity of heritage and language presents greater difficulties in communication and a wider range of needs. Since the mother tongues of the women are so varied, and since those with English as a second language are usually eager to improve their fluency, all the groups are conducted in English with repetition, gesture, and humor filling in the gaps.

As the name "Preparing for Change" implies, the group's purpose is to enable the participants to make significant and lasting changes in their lives. The long-term goals set by the women are individually chosen, e.g., enrolling in education and training to get a job in electronics, joining a community group that is working on local drug problems, taking an abusive husband to court, and joining a support group for battered women. The problem situations that are being addressed are more than individual, however, and their resolution frequently involves joining forces with others. As Burstow (1992) writes, "personal problems are both created and exacerbated by societal power imbalances. Correspondingly, helping women make the connections and resist is key to what feminist counselling is about" (p. 40).

The change process must take place along several axes simultaneously if it is to have an impact on problem situations that are usually long-standing, multidimensional, and maintained by current power structures. It must enable women to make changes at cognitive, emotional, and behavioral levels and to initiate action in the individual or the collective realm. A group offers the ideal vehicle for this endeavor since its dual focus (person/environment) encompasses both the individual and social functioning needs of its members (Alissi, 1981). Moreover, the group process itself offers the well-documented benefits of reducing stigma and social isolation (Gitterman, 1989), developing a democratic mutual aid system (Glassman and Kates, 1990), and providing a forum to try out new roles and behaviors (Middleman and Goldberg, 1988).

As well as identifying and working on the societal barriers facing the participants, the Opportunity for Advancement model builds on the traditional relational strengths of women and develops new ones. As Lewis (1992) writes: "the small social group . . . gives promise of developing the full range of human potential, not discarding spirituality, nurturance or emotion, but adding capacities for assertiveness, conflict resolution, decision making, cooperation and accomplishment of important social (public) tasks" (p. 277). The "Preparing for Change" group incorporates many of the these elements in a structured program that consists of four components:

1. Helping the group to form/creating safety and trust;
2. Validating personal experiences/developing a structural perspective;
3. Learning/sharing new information and skills;
4. Creating a long-term plan for change/ending the group.

This sequence is complementary to the stages of group development that have been identified in the social group work literature, i.e., pre-affiliation, power and control, intimacy, differentiation, and separation (Garland, Jones, and Kolodny, 1978). The area that requires particular balancing, however, given the diversity of the women in the groups, is that of intimacy versus differentiation. The worker must help the group identify common themes and interests and, at the same time, resist the tendency for important differences to be glossed over or minimized. This is critical not only with respect to group functioning but as an experience of building community that women can use in the broader social system. As Lorde (1984) explains, "It is not our differences which separate women, but our reluctance to recognize those differences and to deal effectively with the distortions which have resulted from the ignoring and misnaming of those differences" (p. 122).

At Opportunity for Advancement, one of the unique and important features of the group work method is the use of a structured program–a series of activities that stimulate discussion, suggest new horizons, encourage the sharing of knowledge, and allow new behaviors to be tested. First, it enables workers to make the best use of the relatively brief time span of the group (14 three-hour sessions over a seven-week period). Alissi and Casper (1985) point to the need for the worker in short-term groups to be clear about purposes and goals, and to focus on content, preparation, and structure to make the best use of time. Careful attention to all these variables in the "Preparing for Change" group accelerates the group process and deepens the level of work that can be undertaken.

More important, the use of specific program activities enables participants to develop a critical awareness of the oppressive conditions of their lives. In this respect there are many parallels between the methodology used in feminist consciousness-raising and in popular education or *conscientizao*. First developed in the 1960s in Brazil by Paulo Freire, this model of political work involving educational action with oppressed people is now being used throughout the world. The key to the process is the dialectical methodology described by Canadian popular educators as "a process of education that starts with the daily experience of people (practice), helps them to critically analyze that experience (theory) so that they can collectively act to change that situation (practice)" (Arnold, Barndt, and Burke, undated).

Both feminist consciousness-raising and popular education make use of what Freire terms "codifications." In Latin America, these were usually pictures or sketches because the majority of learners were illiterate, but in current Canadian practice they may include story writing, skits, murals, songs, or human sculptures (Neighborhood Action, 1985). These codifications, usually referred to in North America as activities or exercises, are based on the concrete, existential reality of the participants and reflect both the aspirations of the people and some of the contradictions inherent in their situations. They serve as a starting point for each participant to tell their version of the situation that is presented. As group members "reconsider," through the "considerations" of others, their own previous "consideration" (Freire, 1970, p. 104), the "decoding" or critical analysis of the situation takes place.

In the "Preparing for Change" group, this methodology is used to examine oppression as it relates to gender, class, and race. The diversity of the women's backgrounds, which initially poses some challenges in creating a sense of "groupness," becomes an explicit and valued resource when it comes to examining the structural issues that define and limit participants' circumstances and life chances.

The exercise, "Grandmother, Mother, and Me," for example, draws on family memories to explore and problematize women's work. In this activity, the women choose a subgroup representing one of the three generations and then respond to questions such as "What kinds of work does she do in and outside the home?"; "How much control does she have over her work?"; and "Does she like her work?" After sharing their various experiences, the women go on to discuss whether women's work has changed, and what has remained the same across the generations and across cultures. What begins as a sharing of individual women's situations can easily become a rich discussion about issues that are common to women at a global level, such as their responsibility for children, the long hours that women work in waged and unwaged labor, or their limited access to education and well-paid employment. The chance to view women's work through different historical and cultural lenses can also challenge participants' assumptions about what women *can* and *should* do.

In another example, "The Hats We Wear," the notion of hats is used as a metaphor for social roles, both chosen and ascribed. Naming the "hats," and discussing their feelings about them, enables the women to unpack the value-laden constructs with which they struggle and which often negatively affect their self-esteem, e.g., "welfare mother" with its connotations of laziness and inadequacy, or "immigrant" which is so often used by the dominant culture to convey disentitlement to jobs or resources. This activity reframes individual attributes as socially derived and helps to reduce stigma and self-blame. At a later point, the women also decide which "hats" they would like to take off or de-emphasize and which new ones they would like to take on. This begins the process of taking back control and exercising choice.

Structured activities have received some criticism from social group workers (Garland, 1992) who have been concerned about the tendency for "programmed exercises" to replace authentic learning and the development of democratic structures in the group. While this is a valid concern, it is important to point out that in a feminist group work model the aim is not to deposit facts or prescribe behavior, but to open up the possibilities for self-defined knowledge and self-directed action. As Freire (1970) warns, "since they represent existential situations the codifications should be simple in their complexity and offer various decoding possibilities in order to avoid the brain-washing tendencies of propaganda" (p. 107).

At Opportunity for Advancement, an exercise called the "Shoulds" provides an example of a simple task that offers a variety of responses and analytical frameworks. The women brainstorm together the expectations they received as small girls, as teenagers, and as adult women from parents, teachers, the media, and cultural and religious institutions. Some expectations and values do vary across cultures–being thin, for example, is not positively regarded in societies where food is scarce–but universal themes and contradictions abound, such as women always caring for others, not having needs of their own, being attractive, not being sexually active, and being the social coordinator in the family.

A second part of this theme involves the women in creating a Bill of Rights for themselves. It includes not only existing legal and civil rights, but the freedoms, choices, and basic resources that they would like to have, and which speak eloquently of their oppressed status. These are some examples from a list of 21 "rights" compiled by a recent group that included women from Grenada, Canada, Somalia, Trinidad, Burma, and Iran. Again, various social and cultural perspectives are evident in the responses and even common concerns are differently experienced:

1. Right to walk down the street, not to be afraid of being hurt or raped;
2. Right to have as many kids as I want–many, few, or none;
3. Right to say no to sex if I am not ready;

4. Right to be treated like a man at work, be taken seriously, no sexist jokes;
5. Right to be paid like a man. This means being paid fairly;
6. Right not to have a boyfriend or not to be married and to feel okay;
7. Right to say no to an arranged marriage;
8. Right to dress as we wish;
9. Right to go to school and be educated;
10. Right to have some help.

In the "Preparing for Change" groups, we are concerned with understanding and working on both the external consequences of oppression and its internal manifestations. Experiences of powerlessness, exclusion, and violence have destructive psychological and emotional effects, particularly when coupled with social isolation. Empowerment involves the ability to act on oppressive situations, to participate in society and to be fully oneself. Wyckoff (1980) expresses this succinctly in two basic equations :

$$\text{Oppression} + \text{Lies} + \text{Isolation} = \text{Alienation}$$
$$\text{Action} + \text{Awareness} + \text{Contact} \rightarrow \text{Power}$$

At the beginning of the group, women commonly describe themselves as "dumb," "useless," or "no good as a parent," and their feelings as "angry at everyone," "hopeless," or "crying all the time." Consciousness-raising work itself reframes issues in ways that reduce feelings of personal inadequacy and guilt; it also lets women know that their responses are "normal" and are shared by others in similar circumstances. Elements of the group process that work directly on feelings of self-esteem and competence include emphasizing women's strengths in having survived and managed under difficult conditions, sharing knowledge and problem-solving together, dealing with difference and conflict successfully, and choosing topics and speakers for the information section of the program.

A key aspect of building self-esteem, and ultimately facilitating change, lies in enabling women to exercise more personal power and control in their lives. In part, this involves examining the way in which women are socialized to minimize and forgo their own needs, and taught that their own fulfillment lies in meeting the needs of others

(Levine, 1982). Since women's caring work is invisible and undervalued, it is often hard for participants to see it as work or to acknowledge the stress of care-giving 24 hours a day with little money and few social supports. Group activities validate these realities, encourage greater self-care, and enable the women to experience asking for what they need in the group. Assertiveness training and role-playing allow participants to practice setting limits with others and advocating for themselves in personal and institutional situations.

Just as women's caring, in its nonreciprocal and self-denying manifestations, has often been a disempowering and debilitating undertaking, it has also been the source of women's strength, underpinning their ability to build connections with one another and their resistance. As Miles (1982) explains, "At the same time as it has oiled the wheels of an oppressive system and eased the lot of our rulers, women's service has kept alive an alternative, and in part subversive, set of values and ways of living life" (p. 220). In groups, socially isolated, disenfranchised women are able to develop intimate connections with one another that foster growth, understanding, and new ways of being. As one of our participants wrote in a note she read out loud to the group:

> Our lives have been touched and changed by this wonderful group of women. How can we explain the tears, the love and laughter we have shared? The tears we cried out to one another to release our inner hurts that had held us hostage within ourselves and brought us pain and sickness for so many years. The memory of everything taught and spoken and the knowledge and wisdom we have acquired we will carry this with us for the rest of our lives and know that we have helped one another to grow and to accomplish the goals that are so important to us in our future lives.

Empowerment, though a popular goal in group work, is a misunderstood and complex undertaking. It involves a theoretical stance that understands the workings of exploitive power relations and the need to make them explicit. It requires an ability to create an environment where differences can be experienced in ways that are affirming for the individual and enlightening for others. And it requires a basic belief in the ability of disenfranchised people to find strength and hope in the communal struggle for social change. We, as social workers, need to be part of this struggle.

REFERENCES

Alissi, A. 1981. "The Social Group Work Method: Toward a Reaffirmation of Essentials." Third Annual Symposium on the Advancement of Social Work with Groups. Hartford, Connecticut.

Alissi, A. and Casper, M. 1985. *Time as a Factor in Groupwork: Time-Limited Group Experiences,* Binghamton, NY: The Haworth Press, Inc.

Armstrong, P. and Armstrong, H. 1987. "Looking Ahead: The Future of Women's Work" in *Feminism and Political Economy,* Luxton, M. and Maroney, H. J. (Eds.), Toronto: Methuen.

Arnold, R., Barndt, D. and Burke, B. Undated manual. *A New Weave: Popular Education in Canada and Central America,* Toronto: Ontario Institute for Studies in Education.

Breton, M. 1992. "Liberation Theology, Group Work, and the Right of the Poor and Oppressed to Participate in the Life of the Community," *Social Work with Groups,* Vol. 15, (2/3), 257-269.

Browne, J., Filger, S., and McDonald, V. 1989. *Preparing for Change: A Group Work Manual,* Toronto: Opportunity for Advancement.

Burstow, B. 1992. *Radical Feminist Therapy,* Newbury Park, CA: Sage.

Carniol, B. 1987. *Case Critical: The Dilemma of Social Work in Canada,* Toronto: Between the Lines.

Dhillon, J., and Walter, L. 1993. *Aftercare for Abused Women: A Preliminary Study and Needs Assessment with a Model for Service in Metro Toronto,* Toronto: Author.

Evans, P. 1991. "The Sexual Division of Poverty: The Consequences of Gendered Caring" in *Women's Caring: Feminist Perspectives on Social Welfare,* Baines, C., Evans, P., and Neysmith, S. (Eds.), Toronto: McClelland and Stewart.

Freire, P. 1970. *Pedagogy of the Oppressed.* New York: The Seabury Press.

Fulani, L. 1987. Introducing remarks. *Women and Therapy: The Politics of Race and Gender in Therapy,* Vol. 6, (4).

Garland, J. 1992. Editorial. In *Social Work with Groups Newsletter,* Vol. 8, No. 2, p. 2.

Garland, J., Jones, H. and Kolodny, R. 1978. "Model for Stages of Development in Social Work Groups," in *Explorations in Group Work: Essays in Theory and Practice.* Boston, MA: Practitioners Press.

Gitterman, A. 1989. "Building Mutual Support in Groups," *Social Work with Groups,* Vol. 12 (2), 5-21.

Glassman, U. and Kates, L. 1990. *Groupwork: A Humanistic Approach.* Columbia, SC: London: Sage.

Goldstein, H. 1973. *Social Work Practice: A Unitary Approach,* University of South Carolina Press.

Government of Ontario. 1988. *Transitions: Report of the Social Assistance Review Committee,* Toronto: Queen's Printer for Ontario.

_____ . 1993. *Turning Point: New Support Programs for People with Low Incomes,* Toronto: Queen's Printer for Ontario.

Langan, M. 1985. "The Unitary Approach: A Feminist Critique" in *Women, the Family and Social Work,* Brook, E. and Davis, A. (Eds.), New York: Tavistock.

Lee, J. 1992. "Jane Addams in Boston: Intersecting Time and Space," *Social Work with Groups,* Vol. 15 (2/3), 7-21.

Lepischak, B. 1992. *Missing the Mark: Women's Services Examine Mental Health Programs for Women in Toronto,* Toronto: Coalition for Feminist Mental Health Services.

Levine, H. 1982. "The Personal is Political" in *Feminism in Canada: From Pressure to Politics,* Miles, A., and Finn, G. (Eds.), Montreal: Black Rose Books.

Lewis, E. 1992. "Regaining Promise: Feminist Perspectives for Social Group Work Practice," *Social Work with Groups,* Vol. 15 (2/3), 271-284.

Loewenstein, S. 1976. "Integrating Content on Feminism and Racism into the Social Work Curriculum," *Journal of Education for Social Work,* 12 (1), 91-96.

Lorde, A. 1984. *Sister Outsider,* Freedom, CA: The Crossing Press.

McNay, M. 1992. "Social Work and Power Relations: Toward a Framework for an Integrated Practice" in *Women, Oppression and Social Work,* Langan, M., and Day, L. (Eds.), London: Routledge.

Middleman, R. and Goldberg, G. 1988. "Toward the Quality of Social Group Work Practice," *Roots and New Frontiers in Social Group Work,* New York: The Haworth Press.

National Council of Welfare. 1993. *Poverty Profile Update for 1991,* Ottawa: Author.

Neighborhood Action. 1985. *Neighborhood Action: Recipes for Change,* Sudbury: Sticks and Stones.

Pincus, A. and Minahan, A. 1973. *Social Work Practice: Model and Method,* Itasca, IL: Peacock.

Statistics Canada. 1992. *Women in Canada–A Statistical Report,* Ottawa: Author.

Ursel, J. 1992. *Private Lives, Public Policy,* Toronto: Women's Press.

Weir, L. 1987. "Socialist Feminism and the Politics of Sexuality" in *Feminism and Political Economy,* Luxton, M. and Maroney, H. J. (Eds.), Toronto: Methuen.

Wyckoff, H. 1980. *Solving Problems Together.* New York: Grove.

Chapter 12

Debriefing Groups for Nurses

Joan K. Parry
Jane Tanner

BACKGROUND AND LITERATURE REVIEW

Each time that social workers, nurses, and other health professionals provide crisis intervention and emotional support to an individual or family who has experienced a death, health professionals also experience the grieving process. When discussing the role of the care giver, Fulton (1979) referred to the care giver as a "surrogate griever." As "surrogate grievers," health professionals may experience not only the emotions associated with the grief–i.e., sadness, anger, guilt–but the episode can also arouse memories and feelings surrounding the care giver's own personal losses.

This emotional reaction may become more stressful when the "surrogate griever" is not aware of its normalcy and places unrealistic expectations on her/himself by believing that feelings are unprofessional, demonstrate weakness, interfere with the crisis intervention, or are not supported by the supervisor of his/her institution. Rando (1984), when discussing nurses' grief reactions, concluded that "when there is a lack of understanding of the necessary mourning and grieving that occur when patients die, care givers may feel that they have somehow failed by experiencing such reactions, when in fact these are completely normal and expected" (p. 437).

This observation is supported by an experience of a social worker in an intensive care nursery at a large medical facility in California following the death of a small baby who had been cared for by the nursing staff for several weeks. After the death of the baby, the social worker recognized that one nurse appeared to be having a particularly difficult time. She had also been aware that the nurse had recently had a miscarriage after many years of infertility. The social worker offered to meet with the nurse for a supportive counseling session. The nurse was receptive to this, but asked that the social worker check with the unit supervisor, as she would need to be replaced by a float nurse for approximately one hour. After approaching the unit supervisor with her request, the social worker became discouraged and disillusioned by the supervisor's response. The supervisor explained that the manpower was not available. When pressured for a more specific reason, she informed the social worker that the nursing staff is "used to the death of infants" and "did not need intervention." She further stated that she "did not mean to sound cold, but that was a fact."

This lack of validation and support creates symptoms which lead to emotional drain, as well as detachment from the patient and his or her family. These emotional consequences interfere with the nurses' personal lives, as well as their care of the patient and the family. The ultimate consequence is breakdown and inability to continue in the field of nursing. One nurse who had cared for a seven-month-old infant was very upset when the child died unexpectedly. When this nurse wrapped the body for the morgue, her own grief was not recognized. This nurse was put on medical leave a few days later and never returned to work. This incident was one of many which were instrumental in the development of an organized intervention to combat the negative consequences of unresolved "surrogate grieving" in order to enhance the nurses' ability to perform their jobs and stabilize their personal lives.

The need for intervention is also supported by the literature on care givers' grief. Rando (1984) states the following: "If her accumulated grief is not worked through, the care giver is every bit as vulnerable to all the malignant sequelae of unresolved grief as in any other individual, who has suffered a loss but failed to complete his grief work" (p. 431). The need is especially recognized when working with the unexpected death of newborns and young infants. Not only is the death of an infant a tragic event, but the crisis intervention particular to the death of a baby requires full involvement with the loss. The nurses, as well as the social worker, cleanse the infant in preparation for the family to hold him. Handprints and footprints are completed, pictures are taken, and hair and other memorabilia are collected. The infant is held by a nurse or social worker when transported to the morgue. Holding a dead baby is an emotionally draining experience for nurse or social worker.

The family may spend hours holding the infant while the nurse cares for the mother's medical needs if she has just given birth. This active involvement in the loss exacerbates the nurse's own grief feelings associated with the loss. But who cares for the nurse? What method of intervention would provide effective and regular support for the nursing staff?

In a study examining causes of stress among nurses, Albrecht (1982) found that nurses who discussed their feelings with coworkers and supervisors had lower stress levels than those who did not. This study suggests that peer support is an effective intervention to combat stress among nurses. In another study evaluating the effectiveness of support groups for health care professionals working with AIDS victims, Grossman and Silverstein (1993) found that "support groups with their focus on awareness, shared experiences, supportive and helping relationships, and the emotional consequences of working with people with AIDS, help health care professionals manage stress and enhance their capacity and effectiveness to work with these clients" (p. 144). The authors concluded that health care professionals who participate in support groups feel supported and less isolated. They suggest that a single-session group modality be used in a hospital setting for education and as a response to crisis (Grossman and Silverstein, 1993).

Group practice with individuals who work in institutions contributes significantly to the constructive carrying out of job functions within the institution. The group is also a powerful influence on the institutional environment of the group, as well as on the external community of each of its individual members (Moore and Starkes, 1992, p. 172). These comments relate directly to the earlier discussion of nurses whose grief was not recognized, one of whom never returned to work.

Although no research could be found to demonstrate the effectiveness of a single-session group to provide intervention to health care professionals after a crisis, in particular a death, there was some literature promoting the use of single-session groups in the hospital setting. Single-session groups (also known as debriefing groups) provide an excellent means of assisting the nursing staff with their grief work after the sudden loss of an infant. In addition, such groups are an educational tool which allows nursing staff to learn the necessity of mourning, as well as their own expectations and limitations when assisting families. Therefore, a debriefing group after a death would provide the needed intervention to facilitate appropriate grieving, reduce staff isolation and stress, and enhance continued patient care. In fact, a permanent support group for people who have lost someone through an unexpected death is a powerful testament to the importance of support and mutual aid to these individuals (Amelio, 1993).

THE INTERVENTION

At San Jose Medical Center, debriefings are held regularly after the death of an infant or child and have been found to be a necessary part of this organization, which has one of the busiest trauma centers in Northern California. The debriefing group creates an opportunity for the nursing staff to express their feelings of grief and distress, and to receive both validation and education with the assistance of an experienced facilitator. The following model offers a standardized format that can be utilized in other settings.

Stage I

Immediately after the crisis intervention is completed for the family, the social worker begins the process of organizing a convenient time and place for the staff to meet. The room used for debriefing is dependent upon the unit in which death has occurred; for example, in ICN it is always the nurses' lounge. The debriefing takes place following the 3:00 p.m. shift change, in order to give all of those involved in the crisis a chance to attend. The group lasts 45 to 60 minutes. The number of members depends upon the particular unit in which the death occurred; for example, a labor-and-delivery death will have five or six members, whereas a pediatric death in the trauma service could be 10 or more, often including physicians. Other staff who have been involved and are still on duty are asked to leave their beepers off so that distractions are minimal. Having the group meet at a regular and expected juncture reduces the stigma attached by making it a part of the crisis intervention.

This group has been meeting for more than two years. There is an assumption that group work is optimally effective when it is *institutionalized* and "when it operates as an integral part of the agency (hospital) mission, culture, structure, and process" (Garland, 1992, p. 91). It is especially important to have the assumption of a need for a group to serve the nursing staff, as nurses have been socialized to believe that by not being strong and by having feelings such as depression, anger, etc., they were being unprofessional (Rando, 1984, p. 431; Vachon, Lyall, and Freeman, 1978).

The facilitator, one of the authors, begins the groups by starting with nonthreatening questions such as, "Where were you in the crisis?"; "What was your job and what do you remember?" This encourages each member of the group to discuss his/her role, and it also assists the member in remembering what he/she was experiencing. It is easier to begin the group process by allowing members to start with what they were *doing* rather that what they were *feeling*. This will help the group members become interactive. The goal of this interactive process is to get to feelings. The worker's authenticity is the principle which lays the foundation for overcoming resistance (Milgram and Rubin, 1992), and overcoming resistance enhances the opportunity to foster interactive discussions of feelings.

Stage II

Once the group members become more comfortable, the group moves toward the stage of intimacy (Berman-Rossi, 1993), and the facilitator will inquire about what the members were thinking and feeling. The members, at this stage of the group, begin to verbalize feelings and share emotions that, under other circumstances, would be very difficult to express. The particular crisis subject to intervention might have triggered memories of previous deaths, including those that have occurred outside of the professional setting. The members and the worker identify their own limitations and learn to accept them. They try to realistically look at what can and cannot be accomplished during this brief intervention. Some of the discussion may focus on countertransference issues. This stage can enhance the members' awareness of their own personal feelings about death.

Stage III

The group moves closer to the stage of differentiation. This is the stage in which "the group is working as a unit, is now at its most mature, productive, and cohesive stage" (Berman-Rossi, 1993, p. 77). Worker and members empower each other as care givers and, therefore, enhance their sense of competence when mutual aid and validation are part of the process. They learn that what they may have thought of as insignificant has actually impacted the family's ability to cope with their loss; for example, when the social worker shares with nurses how much the family appreciated the extra support and time they gave to their dying relative, the nurses feel appreciated. They learn about each other's limitations and personal losses in the group, which allows them to ask for and receive help without guilt during a crisis situation. For example, learning that a nurse had recently miscarried and did not feel able to prepare an infant would allow another member to do that part of the intervention. This provides for the uniqueness of each member to be incorporated into group life and thus provides for individual need satisfaction for members (Berman-Rossi, 1993). It also allows for helping members to feel the strength of being "helpers" for more needy members.

The group members may have suggestions on how to reduce stress and how to solve problems during a particular part of the crisis intervention. During one debriefing group after a stillbirth, the nursing staff discussed how to put closure on the procedure of viewing an infant that had continued longer than was considered "healthy" in the grief process. The social worker had left before the parents had completed the viewing of their dead child, and they had held the baby in their hospital room until the next morning, approximately 16 hours. The nursing staff became distressed over the natural decay that takes place if the baby is not placed in the hospital morgue. They all felt unsure of how to proceed.

The above is supported by Barton (1977) when he states, "The lack of shared support and a setting for the expression of feelings in the caregiving milieu may lead to a painful state of isolation, mean-inglessness, and despair" (p. 82).

Stage IV

When closing the group, it is very helpful to discuss what happened to the family after the members ended their contact. The social worker usually stays with the family until they leave. This might have occurred after the nursing staff changed shift. In this situation, the debriefing would take place on the next day. They might want to know what happened to the baby. Was a funeral planned? Did the family invite the staff? Often the family asks the social worker to thank the nursing staff for their assistance and will specifically mention how it helped them.

During this final phase, which is known as separation, "the group must evaluate its work, define any remaining tasks, and realistically attend to whatever is still possible" (Berman-Rossi, 1993, p. 79). In handling this stage, the facilitator can bring closure by using an exercise; for example, she could ask the members to write down the strongest and most uncomfortable feeling that persists, then have the member crumble it up and throw it away.

Lastly, the facilitator can give resources for those individuals who need additional assistance. After a debriefing session, co-workers are more aware of the need to support each other, and consequently, the support continues on a regular basis. Mutual aid is thus continued outside the formal group, and this stage can also be conceptualized as a transition from one group to the next group.

CONCLUSION

The death of a baby or small child is a traumatic event. The ability of nurses and social workers to continue providing support and sympathy to the parents and family is emotionally demanding work that requires intervention in order to avoid overwhelming stress or emotional withdrawal. Group work is very frequently the intervention which provides the help for clients and staff. The debriefing group held within hours after a fetal or infant death is an excellent way to respond to the needs expressed by parents and nursing staff.

REFERENCES

Albrecht, T. (1982). What job stress means for the staff nurse. *Nursing Administration Quarterly, 7*(1), 1-19.

Amelio, R. C. (1993). An AIDS bereavement support group: One model of intervention in a time of crisis. *Social Work with Groups, 16*(1/2), 45-54.

Barton, D. (1977). *Dying and death.* Baltimore, MD: William and Wilkins.

Berman-Rossi, T. (1993). The tasks and skills of the social worker across stages of group development. *Social Work with Groups, 16*(1/2), 69-81.

Fulton, R. (1979). Anticipatory grief, stress, and the surrogate griever. In J. Tache, H. Selye, & S. Day (Eds.), *Cancer, stress, and death.* New York: Plenum.

Garland, J. A. (1992). Developing and sustaining group work services: A systemic and systematic view. *Social Work with Groups, 15*(4), 89-98.

Grossman, A. H., & Silverstein, C. (1993). Facilitating support groups for professionals working with people with AIDS. *Social Work, 38*(2), 144-151.

Milgram, D., & Rubin, J. S. (1992). Resisting resistance: Involuntary substance abuse group therapy. *Social Work with Groups, 15*(1), 95-110.

Moore, E. E., & Starkes, A. J. (1992). The Group-in-institution as the unit of attention: Recapturing and refining a social work tradition. *Social Work with Groups, 15*(2/3), 171-192.

Rando, T. A. (1984). *Grief, dying, and death.* Champagne, IL: Research Press Company.

Vachon, M. L. S., Lyall, W. A. L., & Freeman, S. J. J. (1978). Measurement and management of stress in health professionals working with advanced cancer patients. *Death Education, 1,* 365-375.

Chapter 13

Group Work with Mothers
of Sexually Abused Children

Patricia A. Joyce

In the past decade's explosion of popular and professional interest in child sexual abuse, mothers of incestuously abused children, until recently, constituted a poorly understood and underserved population. Theoretical and clinical formulations about mothers were based on poor research carried out within a patriarchal system which attacked and blamed mothers for the offenders' crimes. Professionals saw mothers as consciously or unconsciously giving consent to the abuse, with their denial of the abuse at disclosure being taken as proof of their "collusion." Because of clinicians' interest in treating incest victims, the treatment of the mother was seen as peripheral to the individual, group, and family treatment of the child victim or the offender.

Over the past five years new studies have appeared examining mothers' personality characteristics and behavior, and effectively challenging collusion as an overarching explanation of the mother's role in the incest scenario (Carter, 1993; Elbow and Mayfield, 1991; Faller, 1988; Gomes-Schwartz et al., 1990; Humphreys, 1992; Myer, 1985; Sirles and Franke, 1989; Wagner, 1991). Most propose group work strategies to address mothers' treatment needs (Damon and Waterman, 1986; Hagood, 1991; Hildebrand and Forbes, 1987; Koch and Jarvis, 1987; Strand, 1990; Strand, 1991; Trepper and Barrett, 1989).

This chapter will present a model for group work practice with mothers of sexually abused children, with a special focus on how group treatment can address the trauma mothers feel upon discovery of their children's molestation.

A review of the treatment literature relating to mothers of sexually abused children will be presented. Common factors of group treatment approaches will be discussed, along with how they differ in addressing mothers' needs.

Also explored will be how group work can help mothers cope with societal role expectations that lead them to be blamed for the abuse. How group work approaches can be particularly helpful in lessening mothers' shame and isolation will be demonstrated through two case examples from the author's practice experience.

REVIEW OF THE TREATMENT LITERATURE

Treatment literature has been somewhat in advance of theoretical writing and research on mothers of sexually abused children, and may have provided a stimulus for research. Within the past few years, clinicians have begun to view mothers as having treatment needs of their own which should be considered in their own right. The theoretical underpinnings of these treatment studies are diverse, but some common factors will be pointed out.

Damon and Waterman's parallel group-treatment model for intra-familially abused preschoolers and their mothers features a directive, structured 13-module therapeutic format, focusing on helping mothers work through their own sexual trauma to aid them in responding appropriately to their children. Themes in each module are drawn from the experience of child victims (Damon and Waterman, 1986, p. 245). They do not attempt to link their treatment model to a conceptualization of mothers of sexually abused children.

Symbiotic relationships between mothers and daughters in father-daughter incest are discussed by Koch and Jarvis (1987), who outline the developmental origin of symbiosis. They posit the mother's treatment needs as crucial to family recovery and prevention of reabuse, and hold that group therapy is the treatment of choice to provide support, lessen social and psychological isolation, as well as to offer appropriate avenues for nurturance, recognition of their own victimization, reduction of dependency, and development of parenting skills (Koch and Jarvis, 1987). Koch and Jarvis offer a less stigmatizing and more psychologically refined viewpoint than previously seen on the mother's role in incestuous families; they connect theory and case examples to group treatment.

Hildebrand and Forbes (1987) present a model of group work with mothers of incestuously abused children based on a family systems approach, but with an acknowledgement of the mothers' self-perception of powerlessness. Giarretto's self-help groups for nonoffending parents and Yalom's conceptualization of the curative factors in group work provide other theoretical influences. Their groups met for 16 weeks and were co-led. They describe stages of group life. They note that 50 to 75 percent of mothers in each group were sexual abuse victims themselves and suffered from traumatic aftereffects. They stress the need to differentiate between treatment needs of mothers of incest victims and mothers of "stranger-abuse" victims. Hildebrand and Forbes conclude that group work can help open up closed family systems and aid in preventing reabuse, and call for "long-term follow-up data" to confirm their "impressions of the effectiveness of groupwork as a major variable in the reduction of further abuse in these families" (p. 303).

In their overall systemic model for incest treatment, Trepper and Barrett (1989) assert that groups for mothers are essential to successful treatment. In groups, anger is a major affective theme–anger at offenders, victims, therapists, and fellow group members. Groups can be especially helpful in aiding members to make important life changes, such as divorcing the offender (p. 229).

Strand (1990) accounts for mothers' behavior using Finkelhor's traumagenic dynamics model for victims of sexual abuse. The four traumagenic dynamics are: sexual traumatization, stigmatization, betrayal, and powerlessness. Strand asserts this model is particularly helpful in assessment and engagement stages of treatment, when losing cases is a risk. In a second paper (1991), she proceeds to explore how each dynamic needs to be addressed during the middle phase of treatment, in which group therapy is the primary modality. Analysis of countertransference reactions is crucial to understanding the difficulties clinicians have in working with these mothers.

Hagood (1991) presents an art therapy group, discussing the themes expressed in mothers' artwork. She holds that the mother's psychological well-being "is essential to the overall treatment of her child" and that mothers are traumatized along with their children (p. 26). Art therapy can draw more members into the group process, can enhance voicing of intense emotions, and can help members provide mutual support. The conceptualization of mothers is based primarily on family systems theory, modified by practice knowledge, and borrowings from codependency literature.

What do these group treatment papers share? Throughout there is a discussion of the mothers' trauma and the impact this has had on reactions to disclosure and relationships with their children. That group work is consistently the treatment of choice indicates clinicians' awareness of mothers' shame and isolation and the need for a supportive atmosphere where they can interact with others with similar experiences. The overall empathic tone of the articles reveals that feminist thought on incest has succeeded in sensitizing workers to mothers. Their differences lie in their theoretical underpinnings and their formats.

THE MOTHERS' GROUP

The group to be presented here originated in a preventive services program within a larger child guidance center in one of the outer boroughs of New York City. Staff at the program had developed a considerable degree of expertise in child sexual abuse treatment, and it was decided that a missing component of the program was a group for mothers of sexually abused children. The group was initiated with the purpose of providing mothers with a time and place of their own where they could meet other women going through similar painful experiences.

Besides starting out with the hunch that a long-term group experience would be most helpful in addressing the deep-seated emotions evoked by the abuse, the leader did not begin with a fully shaped model. Much of what became the model developed out of the group's first few months. Recruiting members for the group was surprisingly easy, and within a few weeks a core group of six women had agreed to attend weekly one-hour sessions. What was striking was how much the mothers in the group differed from so many descriptions of mothers in the therapeutic literature, which portrays them as "hostile and frigid . . . passive and subservient in relation to their husbands" (Vander Mey and Neff, 1986, p. 71). All the members were employed full-time, supporting their families as well as taking responsibility for bringing their victimized children to therapy. They were eager to hear about each other's problems, and eager to offer advice and suggestions on how to maneuver their way through the maze of court hearings and child protective proceedings. Hardly a passive group.

More troubling were the traumatic aftereffects of the abuse the mothers were feeling. Several may have met the diagnostic criteria for posttraumatic stress disorder as defined in the DSM-III-R. Among the symptoms reported were: dreams about the abuse, intrusive recollections of it, sleep and appetite disturbances, loss of concentration, and angry, irritable outbursts.

Interfering with their attempts to begin to work through the trauma was the intense shame and isolation the mothers felt about the molestation. Most reported that they could not confide in any friends or family members, and felt totally alone with their swirling feelings. One member reported driving to a different supermarket so she could avoid neighbors' questions about where her husband had disappeared to. Another mother, whose husband had been sentenced to eight years in prison for raping her two daughters, moved to a completely new neighborhood, at considerable cost and disruption.

Most group members were quite vocal about how blamed and stigmatized they felt by police, child welfare workers, and other professionals. At length they spoke about how painful it felt to find out about their children's abuse, and then to be told they must have or should have known about it in the first place.

The group leader took these issues–trauma, shame and isolation, and societal role expectations–as the ones to address over the course of the group's life. In retrospect it was productive to begin the group without too detailed an agenda, and to allow the group members themselves to develop themes. Such an approach is in accord with sensitive group work practice (Shulman, 1992). Had the worker started out with the idea of moving the mothers toward stronger belief in their children's assertions or toward less antagonistic relations with their children (two legitimate goals in treating mothers of sexually abused children), the mothers might have sensed that they were again being somehow blamed, and might not have made a commitment to the group.

ADDRESSING THE IDENTIFIED ISSUES

Once the worker had identified the issues of trauma, shame and isolation, and societal role expectations, she then had to attend to them in the group context. Because of the group members' previous experiences of feeling condemned by professionals, she decided to adopt as supportive and nonconfrontive a stance as possible. It took some effort to maintain this stance in the face of the anger felt by many group members, who often were court-mandated into treatment, and who viewed the group leader as another potential condemner.

Several mothers at times presented as unconnected and unattuned to their children's emotional and developmental needs. It was tempting to intervene and attempt to redirect their attention to their children. However, after consultation and much thought, it was decided that such a therapeutic strategy could backfire, and be experienced by a mother as another attack on her already damaged sense of competence as a parent. Instead, it was decided to slowly and patiently work in the here-and-now, allow the group process to develop, and to use supportively formulated process comments as a technique (Yalom, 1985). Bit by bit, in small, incremental pieces, the group members themselves laboriously worked on their own pain and confusion.

The nature of the mothers' trauma began to reveal itself, and to reveal a reason why some mothers appeared unattuned to their children. First, the discovery of the abuse, if previously unknown to their own consciousness (as was the case for all but one of the group members), was a traumatic blow. It often involved the loss of financial support and a significant relationship if the offender was a husband or boyfriend. Moreover, the mother was traumatized by the blow to her positive sense of self as a parent, i.e., capable, empathically attuned, able to protect her child. She was revealed to at least part of the world as deficient in a role which in a major way defined her sense of who she was, and this narcissistic injury was experienced as traumatic, and rendered her less able to fulfill her parental function.

Over time it became clear that the traumatization of these mothers was multidetermined. Many, if not most of them, carried histories of prior trauma. Some reported having been sexually abused themselves.

Many had been traumatized by battering, alcoholism, drug abuse, and physical abuse in their families of origin or by their partners.

As the mothers in the group felt themselves listened to, supported, and not condemned by one another and by the group leader, some of them spoke of how traumatization had at times interfered with their capacity to respond with full support and belief to their children's allegations. Several spoke of feeling "frozen" and unable to feel.

THE GROUP AND THE LEADER

Even though the leader made efforts to distinguish herself from other professionals who had negatively assessed the mothers' behavior and attitudes, it was inevitable that at certain points in the life of the group the members viewed her as someone whose rules they needed to break. About six months into the course of the group, there was an intensely charged session in which the mothers dwelt at length on what punishments they would like to inflict on the abusers. After the usual ending discussion, the leader left the group room, assuming the members would shortly go out one by one, as had been their habit. It was surprising to return about 30 minutes later to discover that all six members were still sitting in the therapy room, deeply absorbed in their rage at the men who had hurt their children. While commenting positively on how strongly they felt committed to the group as a place where they could safely let such feelings out, the leader explained that the office was now closing (it was very late), and they would have to leave. Though the members complied, several commented that they did not understand why they could not continue the discussion. The worker replied that it would be a great topic to talk about in the next meeting.

Reflection upon this incident made it clear that several factors contributed to its occurrence. One was that the worker had failed to understand how heavily charged the group's content had been—one member talked about how she wanted to put a blowtorch to the offender's genitals. With more awareness, the leader might have spent more time helping the members process and reflect on how raw their feelings were. Not giving the group the opportunity to do so meant they had to spend more time on their own trying to understand what had happened in their own way. Another factor was that the group had achieved enough cohesiveness to be able to mount a challenge to the leader's authority about when the group ended. Yet another factor involved the mothers seeing the worker as a representative of all the people in their past who had not met their needs, who had not given them enough, and who then told them they could not do what they wanted.

In the next session the worker brought up how the group had continued beyond its usual time. With one week to cool off the participants could reflect on how scary the feelings they expressed had been, and how they felt they needed more time to talk through what they were feeling. One member was even able to touch on how her "annoyance" at the worker reminded her of how she used to feel when her mother told her to get off the telephone. In retrospect the incident was extremely fruitful, and moved the group members on to further levels of self-examination.

IMPACT OF THE GROUP:
TWO CASE EXAMPLES

Betty: Reconceptualizing Denial

Betty, a 31-year-old married mother of two daughters, employed as a night nursing supervisor at a large hospital, was referred to the clinic along with her 12-year-old daughter, Kristen, after Kristen disclosed that her father had sexually abused her. The abuse involved oral sex, and Kristen stated that her father had never threatened her. Betty was stunned and disbelieving, especially since the entire family had been in family therapy for two years, after Kristen previously disclosed that her father had molested her. The husband denied the new allegations. Despite her disbelief, Betty immediately threw her husband out of the home and called child protective services. She called the family therapist and told him she would seek treatment elsewhere.

Betty herself was the victim as a child of repeated brutal rapes by her alcoholic father; her own mother never believed her, and Betty stopped the abuse by physically attacking her father and running away to her maternal grandparents home, where she spent the rest of her adolescence.

By the time Betty began in the group, she said with great distress and anger that she felt helpless, that she "had to believe her daughter" even though it seemed impossible. She reported insomnia and nightmares.

Betty was at a level of belief often seen in mothers of molested children when they first come for treatment. She had some cognitive belief, but emotionally could not integrate this belief with what she knew of her husband. This stage might be called denial, but only if denial is conceptualized as an expected part of the difficult and painful process of trying to understand the abuse, a process all mothers of sexually abused children struggle with. In the group she frequently acted as a cotherapist or "internal leader," actively seeking out from fellow mothers how they were coping with their children's victimization (Shulman, 1992, p. 318).

To assist Betty in dealing with her so-called "denial," the worker had to, in Shulman's terms, "synthesize support and demand," which can only be done effectively when the worker is aware of her own feelings and capable of managing them effectively (Shulman, 1992, p. 374). Here the leader had to strive to understand both the dilemma that the abuse placed Betty in, as well as the leader's own wish for Betty to believe her daughter fully and completely. Moreover, the leader realized that she had bought into the societal expectations placed on mothers of sexually abused children: that they should somehow have known about the abuse, despite the abuser's capacity to enforce secrecy. These expectations are a natural outgrowth of the societal double bind all mothers are placed in. They are the recipients of an extremely subtle, yet intensely disempowering, double message: know and be responsible for everything related to your children, despite the fact that as women you are denied access to the economic and social powers that could most influence outcomes in their lives. The worker was able to use this understanding in the group to help Betty integrate the clashing beliefs, and eventually move to a level of deeper belief in and empathy with her daughter.

The group members pointed out how she seemed to expect Kristen to respond to her molestation in the same way that Betty had dealt with her own, despite the tremendous differences between the two situations. After somewhat more than nine months in the group, Betty announced that she now felt that everything Kristen had alleged was true, and she began to display much more warmth and affection when talking about her daughter.

Gina: The "Crazy" Mother

> Gina, a 36-year-old divorced mother of one son, Ben, aged 5, self-referred to the clinic, stating that her ex-husband, who was suing for custody, had sexually molested the boy. Gina worked in sales. Her husband had abandoned them for another woman about two years earlier, and Gina alleged that the abuse had occurred during a weekend visit. Ben, who had just started kindergarten, was completely out of control there, and the teacher was pushing for a special education evaluation. Ben was completely silent about the allegations, with his mother explaining that he would speak only to her about it, and indicating that she believed "much more had gone on" than he would talk about. Gina had been physically abused by her father, a compulsive gambler, who also beat her mother. Both her parents had recently died.
>
> In the group Gina talked loudly and incessantly, sometimes verging on incoherence, frequently interrupting other mothers. She thought of the clinic as a place where she could get help in proving the allegations against her husband.

Initially, Gina appeared to be what Shulman terms a "deviant member" of the group (Shulman, 1992, p. 205). The worker questioned whether she could continue in the group at all. After several weeks, however, the worker was able to point out how Gina's agitation may have been speaking for some feelings other members had, but were not just then able to express. After this Gina began to listen to the other members' concerns with fewer interruptions. She began to hear the suggestions other mothers made about how to deal with her custody battle with her ex-husband. Slowly she began to present herself as less "crazy" and as more in pain and deeply concerned for her son's welfare. She spoke of how alone she felt because of the abuse, and of how she had no one she could talk to about it. It became clear that Ben had tentatively disclosed some kind of molestation to her, and that this traumatic revelation had split her world apart, reawakening old traumas she was ill-equipped to handle, given her recent losses of husband and parents. She became more attuned to Ben's developmental needs, and worked actively with the school to help him adjust there.

Gina always saw both the group and the agency primarily as vehicles to help her in her battle with her ex-husband. Even though this was not in line with how the worker saw her need for services, it did meet an important need for Gina. Getting this need taken care of in group freed Gina to be able to give more to her son, even though her perception of the purpose of the group differed from the worker's.

CONCLUSION: IMPLICATIONS FOR PRACTICE

This chapter has presented a group for mothers of sexually abused children, exploring how group methods can be particularly helpful in addressing the three issues of traumatization, shame and isolation, and societal role expectations. These issues developed out of the material the mothers brought to the group themselves. The focus of other groups of mothers might well be different, but given the recent new research on these mothers, it is likely that these three themes would crop up at some time in the life of most groups for mothers of molested children.

It is important to note that the mothers discussed here are not representative of the population of all mothers of sexually abused children. Mothers who seek treatment, or who comply with court-mandated treatment, may be more likely to believe their children at disclosure, and may be more amenable and open to intervention. Still, it is hoped that the experience presented here can add to the current revision, and help mitigate the pervasiveness of the collusion hypothesis. Because they build on clients' innate capacities, group work techniques are particularly suited to working with mothers of sexually abused children. Such techniques need to be constantly refined and evolved to meet the treatment needs of these much-maligned women.

REFERENCES

Carter, B. (1993). Child sexual abuse: Impact on mothers. *Affilia, 8*(1), 72-90.

Damon, L. and Waterman, J. (1986). Parallel group treatment of children and their mothers. In K. McFarlane et al. (Eds.), *Sexual abuse of young children*. New York: Guilford, 244-298.

Elbow, M. and Mayfield, J. (1991). Mothers of incest victims: Villains, victims, or protectors? *Families in Society: The Journal of Contemporary Human Services, 72*(2), 78-86.

Faller, K. C. (1988). The myth of the "collusive mother." *Journal of Interpersonal Violence, 3*(2), 190-196.

Gomes-Schwartz, B., Horowitz, J. M., Cardarelli, A. P., Salt, P., Myer, M., Coleman, L., and Sauzier, M. (1990). The myth of the mother as "accomplice" to child sexual abuse. In Gomes-Schwartz, B. Horowitz, J. M., and Cardarelli, A. P. (Eds.), *Child sexual abuse: The initial effects.* (pp. 109-131). Newbury Park, CA: Sage.

Hagood, M. M. (1991). Group art therapy with mothers of sexually abused children. *The Arts in Psychotherapy, 18*, 17-27.

Hildebrand, J. and Forbes, C. (1987). Group work with mothers whose children have been sexually abused. *British Journal of Social Work, 17*, 285-304.

Humphreys, C. (1992). Disclosure of child sexual assault: Implications for mothers. *Australian Social Work, 45*(3), 27-35.

Koch, K. and Jarvis, C. (1987). Symbiotic mother-daughter relationships in incest families. *Social Casework, 68*(2), 94-101.

Myer, M. (1985). A new look at mothers of incest victims. *Journal of Social Work and Human Sexuality, 3*, 47-58.

Shulman, L. (1992). *The skills of helping individuals, families, and groups*. Itasca, IL: F. E. Peacock.

Sirles, E. A. and Franke, P. J. (1989). Factors influencing mothers' reactions to intrafamily sexual abuse. *Child Abuse and Neglect, 14*, 129-139.

Strand, V. C. (1990). Treatment of the mothers in the incest family: The beginning phase. *Clinical Social Work Journal, 18*(4), 353-366.

_____ . (1991). Mid-phase treatment with mothers in incest families. *Clinical Social Work Journal, 19*(4), 377-389.

Trepper, T. and Barrett, M. J. (1989). *Systemic treatment of incest*. New York: Brunner/Mazel.

Vander Mey, B. J. and Neff, R. L. (1986). *Incest as child abuse: Research and applications*. New York: Prager.

Wagner, W. G. (1991). Depression in mothers of sexually abused vs. mothers of nonabused children. *Child Abuse and Neglect, 15*(2), 99-104.

Yalom, I. (1985). *The theory and practice of group psychotherapy*. New York: Basic Books.

Chapter 14

Sexual Offenders Group Treatment: The ESAT Experience in Toronto, Canada

Kalev Helde

It was primarily during the 1980s that practitioners began to recognize that adolescents are capable of committing sexual offenses. Work being done with adult sexual offenders was finding that a large number of self-reports admitted to this behavior having started as early as age 12. This is the same era when sexual victimization was being recognized. In the late 1970s, adult women who began to disclose sexual abuse indicated that frequently the victimization had occurred when they were children. The feminist movement allowed these individuals to tell their stories and the helping professions began to realize that if these women had been sexually abused in the past as children, sexual abuse among the current generation of children was probably happening as well.

Anecdotal information about adolescent sexual offending began to be viewed differently by both human services professionals and the criminal justice system. In the past such reports were treated quite lightly–the adolescent was curious about sex; there was a desire to experiment; "he's maturing too quickly;" and it was sexual play. It was assumed that a good chat between the parent and child, or two or three appointments with a counselor would solve the problem, and the adolescent would abandon this wanton curiosity and defer sexual activity until age of majority and with a consenting age mate. But researchers began to find it was not so straightforward.

In the various areas of dysfunctional or aberrant behavior, self-reporting by offenders is the most unreliable. Healthy sexuality is seldom discussed openly; it is far less likely that anyone would admit to inappropriate sexual behavior.

In a study of 411 perpetrators, Abel, Mittleman, and Becker (1986) found that the onset of deviant arousal before the age of 15 occurred in 42 percent of their subjects. And in 57 percent of the sample, deviant arousal had begun by the age of 19. Breaking their sample further into assault characteristics, the authors found that among homosexual pedophiliacs, 53 percent reported the onset of deviant arousal before the age of 15 years and 74 percent before 19 years of age. Their article also notes that self-reporting by offenders is unreliable because of their high level of denial.

These researchers also found that on average an adult sexual offender admitted to 581 attempted sexually inappropriate behaviors and 533 completed offenses. The average number of victims per offender was 336. It was also found that among this adult population, the average career in sexual offending had lasted 12 years before any intervention occurred, whether through the criminal justice system or clinical treatment. Thus, 44 victims a year per offender would have been involved. The majority of victims (56 percent) were under the age of 14; another one-third of the victims were between 14 and 17 years of age.

To add to these figures, Becker, Cunningham-Rathner, and Kaplan (1986) found in research on rape that 21 percent of all forcible rapes committed in the United States in 1978 were carried out by males in the 13 to 18 age group. Their study did not touch upon other pedophiliac behaviors.

In other research on adolescent offenders, Fehrenbachr et al. (1986) found that of 305 subjects, the average age of the adolescent offender was 14.8, and of this group 57.6 percent had committed at least one other sexual offense prior to the current disclosure. This sample group also included eight young females who had been involved in sexually abusive behavior. Fehrenbach et al. found social isolation to be the most significant characteristic of the adolescent offenders they studied. Most of this sample group could not clearly identify any friendships. The role of family dynamics was also found to impact significantly on incidents of adolescent sexual offending.

Preliminary research by J. Worling at the Thistletown Regional Center in Toronto (Worling and Berry, 1990), in a program that works with sexual abuse in the family, has also highlighted some of the characteristics of adolescent sexual offenders. Worling studied

30 adolescent male sex offenders, aged 13 to 19 years, who entered treatment programs. His findings show these young men demonstrate characteristics that include:

- Minimal empathy, frequent failure to take the perspective of others before acting or making decisions;
- High levels of alcohol use, but not significant drug use;
- Extremely high levels of satisfaction with respect to feelings of masculinity;
- Highly conservative attitudes toward sexuality;
- Endorsement of myths about rape (e.g., she wanted it);
- Harboring of a great deal of resentment toward others, along with projection of hostility in the form of suspicion;
- Social reticence and nonassertiveness;
- High impulsivity and willingness to engage in risk-taking behaviors;
- Difficulty in accepting responsibility for their actions and loose ethical boundaries;
- Preference to deal with tangible and concrete tasks as opposed to abstractions;
- Low feelings of self-esteem;
- High levels of familial marital discord, isolation from the community, and unfair parental discipline;
- Difficulties with peers.

Metropolitan Toronto has a population of about three million people, yet only a handful of organizations offer treatment programs for young sexual offenders. As a dysfunctional population group, they are hard to engage in therapy, but more so, they appear to be a group that is rejected by many professionals. Their victims tend to be younger siblings, close family friends, or persons from babysitting arrangements. Their offenses are viewed as distasteful and a strong sense of denial pervades social work practice in their regard.

The Etobicoke Adolescent Offenders Group is an offshoot of the Etobicoke Sexual Abuse Treatment (ESAT) Program. ESAT represents a cooperative effort of a number of social services agencies in the Metropolitan Toronto suburb. Groundwork for the organization began in 1988, and in the fall of 1989 the first referrals were accepted. Two child protection agencies, several children's mental health centers, residential settings, and counseling agencies contribute social workers' work time to become involved in the project. The first groups offered were for teen victims of sexual abuse, latency age boys and girls, and a mums and tots group. A mothers' group commenced in January 1990. As one of the needs expressed by the community was for more resources into treatment for adolescent sexual offenders, ESAT undertook to provide this service as well. The group is co-led by two therapists with child welfare backgrounds and years of experience working in the area of sexual abuse and with alleged offenders directly. Having a male-female partnership to co-lead this group was seen as being more effective than same-sex therapists. In this way male/female role differences, values, and expectations could be handled in a more objective manner.

After several months of planning, readings, training opportunities, and consultation with other professionals already offering adolescent offender groups in the city, the first pregroup interviews took place in the fall of 1990, with the group scheduled to start that October.

The adolescent offenders group offered by ESAT is open to males between the ages of 13 to 18 who have acknowledged responsibility or at least participation in a sexual offense. Referrals are accepted from social service agencies across Toronto, but primarily from the west end suburbs. It is mandatory that the child continues to have a case manager at the referring agency to serve as a liaison with the family or caretaker, and to provide individual intervention as deemed necessary by the ESAT group leaders.

Prior to acceptance into the group, the child and his caretakers must have attended at least one pregroup interview to assess suitability, motivation, and commitment to the program. Also, each referred young man is required to complete a battery of psychosocial testing conducted by staff at the Thistletown Regional Center. It is preferred that the testing be concluded prior to admission into the group; however, in many situations, it can be carried on concurrently. Only in cases where the pregroup interviews are not conclusive is inclusion into the group deferred until the test results can provide clearer information about the child as an offender.

At the pregroup interviews, the child is asked to describe the nature of his sexual offenses, to suggest some ideas why he may benefit from the treatment, and, together with his parent or caretaker, to provide a social history, as well as information about his knowledge of sexuality and sexual development. Adolescents admitted into the ESAT program may have been involved in the criminal justice system as a result of their sexual offending; however, many have not been charged with any offense.

ESAT offender group meetings are held weekly, each session being 90 minutes. The group meets from mid-October to early June, with occasional breaks to coincide with school holidays. It is emphasized with the families that most offender treatment groups are long-term and that successful completion of such a program will require from 18 to 24 months. It is also stressed that virtually no excuse is acceptable for nonattendance.

To maintain some continuity and cohesion in light of the extensive summer break, the group leaders have proposed to its membership that monthly meetings be planned from June to September. These are not working sessions, but rather take the form of film nights or possible outings to promote social skills among the adolescents.

To plan and operate a sexual offenders group, practitioners must abandon many of their conventional group work intervention skills. It is thought that in work with sexual offenders, concepts such as empathy, support, and client self-determination do not work. These are seen as manipulative devices that offenders utilize to gain the confidence and complicity of their sexual victims. One expert in work with sexual offenders, J. Ross, suggests that the group leaders must be confrontational and work toward the erosion of clients' highly developed denial and justification mechanisms (Loss and Ross, 1988). Offenders portray a great deal of self-pity and tend to place the responsibility of the offenses on their victims (e.g., she could have said no; she should have told me to stop).

Four major components characterize the ESAT offenders group model. First, during the course of treatment, the participants must acknowledge their offense(s) in explicit detail. Second, they need to take responsibility for their actions, acknowledging that the victim was the one victimized and that the offender's action was entirely his own doing. Third, group members need to develop empathy for their victims and devise ways in which they might relate to the assault victims. Finally, the adolescents need to recognize the factors and events which led to their offending, and devise new patterns of behavior and coping that do not include sexual victimization.

Upon admission to the offenders program, members are advised that treatment may be up to two years; however, graduation is possible at the end of a 26-week cycle. The significant areas to be covered during this time are victim empathy, personal responsibility, sex education, and an understanding of the sexual offending cycle, which includes steps to be taken to break the cycle. Collateral areas that are covered include development of more appropriate social skills, anger control, recognition of one's own victimization, and enrichment of self-esteem and self-concept.

Group work appears to work more effectively with this client population than individual therapy. When the sexually offending behavior has been disclosed and the adolescent confronted with the truth, he goes through a period of self-remorse and self-pity. He tends to perceive himself as a victim of the investigation. In the group setting, the offender continues to be confronted by the inappropriateness of his behavior, but he receives solace and support from the other group members. No longer is he an isolated aberration of sexual dysfunction; rather, he is just like the other adolescents in the room.

Inevitably the group members establish an internal hierarchy. There is a sense of awe when it is learned that someone may have had several victims, or that one boy carried out penal penetration whereas others may have been disclosed for fondling or other seemingly less serious offenses.

It is a learning process during the first few weekly sessions. Experiences in the court system are compared. Some may have been charged with sexual assault and found guilty. Others may have merely been cautioned by local police. It becomes the group leaders' task to moderate such comparisons and offer some explanations for the inequities of the legal system. Whether the offenses were committed against male or female victims may become an issue. It is a perception held by most adolescents that sexual involvement with another male denotes homosexuality and this misconception needs to be explained by group leaders.

In individual therapy, adolescents feel a sense of guilt and embarrassment in admitting to their sexual behavior and sexual practices.

Despite the therapist's reassurances that sexual fantasies are quite normal or that virtually everyone has masturbated some time in their lives, sexual taboos make it difficult for teenagers to divulge this information to an adult. Yet in the group setting, there is more freedom for this type of dialogue. There are usually a few members who are more open to discussing these areas and they serve as a catalyst for the members who have difficulty opening up.

In other group work settings, a certain amount of collusion exists among members. If a participant is reticent or closed, the group tends to protect that individual and may even state that "he is not yet ready." Offenders give their group colleagues little opportunity to become ready. In an effort to maintain control, they will be more confrontational and place significant pressure on those who are not participating at the same level. This may be learned from the group leaders' practice as well. Rather than wait for the adolescents to volunteer responses or impressions, the group leaders will call upon them by name or establish a sequence for reporting back. Usually the teenagers determine their own sequence, whether by age, time of arrival, or alphabetically.

The first weeks of the program are primarily educational, although the introduction of topics and issues fluctuates throughout the year. The ESAT model views sex education as an important factor in successful completion of the program. It is surprising to find that offenders are generally very naive and uninformed about sexual issues.

Useful tools to develop discussion are various paper and pencil exercises. Questions asked reflect a range of sexual myths and misconceptions. Most myths tend to be endorsed by the boys and discussion frequently yields new insight into the issues. Another exercise which proves to be popular is referred to as "sex words." A collection of about 40 index cards is dealt to the group members, including the co-leaders. Each card has printed on it a word or short phrase related to sexuality or sexual interaction. In turn, each participant is asked to define one of his cards, or if unsure, to request clarification from the rest of the group.

Pertaining to healthy sexuality and to social skills, an individual session can be spent discussing how to meet girls or how to ask them on a date. As with all the topics covered through the ESAT group, no issue is totally resolved during the course of one or two sessions. There is a lot of repetition, reconnecting, and reexamination. Comments made during a discussion on dating will inevitably be reintroduced several months later, possibly when the group is dealing with sexual fantasies or victimization.

In the first sessions of a new cycle, each group member is required to give a statement of his sexual offending. The information must include the ages, names, and relationships of the victims, a description of the abuse, and information about events preceding the first incident. This discussion usually includes the process that led to the victim's disclosure and the ensuing investigation. Giving the adolescents an opportunity to ventilate about having been found out is a cathartic process and is one of the first steps to expressing individual feelings. Embarrassment, anger, guilt, and injustice are some of the emotions they go through immediately after being confronted with their victims' allegations.

Hearing the self-disclosures leads into an exercise of defining sexual offending. Rape and sexual contact with younger children are easily identified by offenders as types of sexual assault. Voyeurism, exhibitionism, pornography, and other hands-off offenses are not as obvious to them, and it is not unusual that much later in the program the group members will allude to such acts having preceded their own hands-on offending behavior.

There are also several exercises that can be introduced to help the offenders become more familiar with types of offending and offender profiles. Scenarios about various offending behaviors give the adolescents a better sense that sexual offending has many facets and that a variety of excuses may be offered. They realize that some aspects of their offending behaviors are not as horrific as those described and this gives them more latitude to speak to their own experiences.

To introduce victim empathy, group leaders again begin with an external approach. The group is asked to think of situations in their own lives where they felt injustices were committed against them. Being wrongfully accused of something at school or by their parents, or being arrested for a friend's shoplifting are some examples of their own victimization. Anger and hostility are the most common emotions associated with these situations. The identification of physical abuse or overdiscipline in the home leads the group closer to victim empathy. Once this concept is fairly well understood by the group, the area of sexual victimization is approached. Here again, some of the offenders may feel comfortable in addressing situations in their own lives where they feel sexual abuse occurred. And when this happens, the balance of the group tends to respond positively and exhibit some level of empathy with that adolescent.

This author has also had opportunities to co-lead a treatment group for adolescent female victims of sexual assault concurrently with the offenders program. The parallels in issues for the two population groups have provided unique intervention techniques. Each group has significant curiosity about the other. The victims express anger that their group leader is even willing to engage with sexual offenders. The perpetrators, on the other hand, reflect a totally inappropriate lascivious interest in meeting the teen victims. An exercise which the victims complete during the last quarter of their treatment program includes the writing of letters to their molesters. With their permission, the letters have been shared with the adolescent offenders.

The letters precipitate genuine anger that these transgressions of trust have occurred. Again the offender will initially externalize the anger, directing it at the parent or uncle who participated in sexual activity with a young girl. It is then an opportunity for the group leaders to draw this issue back to the group members as to whether their offenses can be perceived any differently from those depicted in the victims' letters. In each case, the victims were well-known to the offenders, some equilibrium of trust existed between them, an established level of authority was violated, and it is the victim who suffered most. Again and again, the group leaders need to confront the members, both individually and as a group, to let them know that their actions were equally devastating to their victims.

In the ESAT model, most weekly sessions introduce a new area to be discussed and understood. If an appreciable amount of work is accomplished the preceding week, exercises can be more relaxed and less participatory. Made-for-television films or weekly television programs provide some appropriate material. "Cagney and Lacey," for example, has an episode where a female police officer is date raped. The focus of the program is the officer's emotional reaction to the violation.

Poster art and collages present modalities to express personal feelings about victimization or they can be a means of expressing group members' perceptions of victims' emotions toward assault. Whenever such modalities are used, the group leaders need to provide the focus and themes of the art work and the members are required to explain the content of their work in subsequent sessions.

An important component of the group treatment model for adolescent offenders is developing an understanding of their own offending behavior. This is perhaps one of the most difficult requirements of the program. As indicated earlier, offenders are more capable of dealing with concrete situations. Hence, working with the use of profiles, stories, or real-life situations flows fairly well. But attaching abstract notions to their offending behavior is an arduous task for the adolescents.

Helping young offenders to recognize and take responsibility for their own offending behaviors is one of the most strenuous tasks of the treatment group. At the time when this demand is made, the participants will have learned a fair amount about their misconceptions, their excuses, and about themselves in general. There is some identification of circumstances in their lives that precipitated their sexually abusive behavior. Thought distortions, also known as thinking errors, tend to be a major stumbling block in their ability to take such responsibility. Excuses they had given earlier for their behavior are reexamined.

The member who claims that he became aroused and wanted sexual activity because a female was wearing a short skirt, for example, is asked to recall whether this was the case with his own five-year-old sister. Similarly, justifying his actions by saying he was also molested by a teenage male when he was four years old is no longer adequate. The group leaders need to be more confrontational and, with the aid of other group members, these individual myths or thought distortions are eroded.

The Mike Tyson rape case proved to be an invaluable modality to provide intervention relating to thought distortions. Originally, several members of the group sided with Tyson, believing his victim was out for money, or that she should not have placed herself in such a vulnerable position with the well-known boxer. An article in Canada's *Globe and Mail* newspaper described Tyson's sentencing hearing and cited several comments that he made before the judge to justify his behavior. At the start of this exercise, the group was asked to reflect on being in the same position before a judge about to pass sentence for sexual assault. It was evident from their responses that some effective listening had occurred in group sessions. Primarily, the group members indicated they would want the judge to know they were sorry, and would want to apologize to the victim. In addition, they said they realized their own responsibility in the act. On the other hand, Mike Tyson attempted to defend himself during his pre-sentence statement to the extent of identifying himself as the victim of the rape incident.

During the course of an eight-month cycle there are two or three opportunities for group members to meet individually with the therapists and their case managers to review progress. Again, they are regularly advised that there are additional issues that may need to be addressed during a second cycle and that the program is not governed by pass or fail grades. Their competency in establishing victim empathy is an important criteria, as is their progress in identifying their own behaviors on the abuse cycle. The group is also given opportunities to evaluate each other. In general, their evaluations are fairly honest and thought out. At this stage of the group process, they are able to accept criticism from their peers and have developed adequate trust with the adults to listen to their comments.

The ESAT adolescent sexual offenders group program entered its fourth year in the fall of 1993. Several current members have returned and there are referrals for new participants. Blending the group in this way can be effective in that the more senior members will be role models for the recruits. The trust and commitment the seniors have established serve as a bridge to the therapists for the new members. In an offenders group, it appears to be easier to accept criticism and direction from one's peers than it is from the professional practitioners.

Current research does not present an optimistic future for adolescent sexual offenders. Recidivism is high, particularly among pedophile offenders. However, the research of Abel, Mittelman, and Becker indicates that most adult sexual offenders began their careers by age 12. Providing treatment for this young client group may at least deter a few teenagers from reoffending. Successful treatment of just one sex offender may well reduce the number of victims astronomically.

REFERENCES

Abel, G. G., Mittelman, M. S., and Becker, J. V. (1986). *Sexual Offenders: Results of Assessment and Recommendations for Treatment.* In Ben-Aron, M. H., Hucker, S. J., Webster, C. D. (Eds.), Clinical Criminology: The Assessment and Treatment of Clinical Behaviour, M and M Graphics and the Clarke Institute of Psychiatry: Toronto, Ont.

Becker, J. V., Cunningham-Rathner, J. and Kaplan, M. S. (Dec. 1986). Adolescent Sexual Offenders, *Journal of Interpersonal Violence,* I (4), pp. 431-445.

Fehrenbach, P. A., Smith, W., Monasterskky, C., and Deisher, R. W. (April 1986). Adolescent Sexual Offenders: Offenders and Offense Characteristics, *American Journal of Orthopsychiat,* 56(2), 225-233.

Loss, P., and Ross, J. E. (1988). Risk Assessment/Interviewing Protocol for Adolescent Sex Offenders, unpublished.

Richardson, J., Loss, P., and Ross, J. E. (1988). Psycho-Educational Curriculum for Adolescent Sex Offenders, unpublished.

Worling, J. R. and Berry, R. E. (March 1990.) Adolescent Sex Offenders: Preliminary Psychometric Data and Implications for Assessment and Treatment, presented at the XXII International Conference on Behavioral Sciences, Banff, Alberta, Canada.

Chapter 15

Effective Treatment Strategies with Adult Incest Survivors: Utilizing Therapeutic Group Work Methods Within the Context of an Immediate Family

Neil Stokes
Judith Gillis

To live, I must have strength
To have strength, I must heal
To heal, I have to be honest
To be honest, I have to feel "safe"

−15-year-old survivor,
Bay St. George, NF

INTRODUCTION

Sexual abuse of children, including incest, exists in most Western societies and transcends all boundaries of race, religion, socioeconomic class, age, and gender. Research has found that sexual abuse has been experienced by 33 percent of all males and 50 percent of all females (Report of the Committee on Sexual Offenses Against Children and Youth, 1984). Statistics from Newfoundland's Department of Social Services reveal that between the years 1981 and 1988/89 the reported cases of child sexual abuse, including incest, rose in excess of 5000 percent (Report of the Archdiocesan Commission of Inquiry into the Sexual Abuse of Children by Members of the Clergy, 1990, pp. 32-33). Research suggests that there is under reporting in all areas of sexual abuse and that the majority of sexual abuse survivors/victims do not seek intervention from public agencies (Report of the Committee, 1984, p. 193). Therefore, the actual number of children and adults affected by sexual abuse and incest is probably higher than the reported rates, so that the needs for intervention services are potentially far beyond current capacities. The predominance and extent of sexual abuse is unlikely to be any different in the rural region of Bay St. George, Newfoundland, the setting for this paper.

COMMUNITY PROFILE AND RESOURCE BACKGROUND

The Bay St. George region is located in western Newfoundland and has a population of approximately 28,000. The town of Stephenville contains about 8,000 people and is the major population center. The rest of the people live in a string of small towns and communities covering a large geographic area encompassing the Port aux Port Peninsula and Bay St. George region. The town of Stephenville itself is a relatively new and cosmopolitan community which was an American air force base during and after World War II. The more isolated communities within this region are for the most part older and homogeneous in nature, with some having a Micmac heritage, some Francophone, and others with English or Scottish backgrounds. The majority of the population in the region is Roman Catholic. The local economy, not unlike that of many rural regions of Canada, is depressed, with employment largely dependent on a single industry (i.e., pulp and paper mill) and the public service sector. In May 1992, multiple adult siblings disclosed incest and extensive physical abuse by their aging father, which resulted in the local police proceeding with criminal charges. These disclosures were prompted by several factors, including heightened public awareness due to a number of high-profile sexual abuse cases, both locally and provincially, involving multiple victims of a single offender. These disclosures, after what had been for most in this family a lifelong silence, precipitated an upheaval and crisis impacting on the immediate and extended family to a degree that all were unable to imagine or comprehend. In the midst of this crisis, eight of the 18 adult siblings requested help from a rural human service system that was not equipped to provide services to such a large number of individuals facing a problem of this magnitude.

Few services were available for an appropriate response to this disclosure by multiple adult sibling incest survivors. The local Women's Center was able to provide support to victims of sexual abuse, but it was not a structured counseling service. The Social Work Department at the regional hospital in Stephenville was primarily responsible for in-patient services, but lacked the resources to respond to sexual abuse survivors/victims in the community. The Mental Health Program at the regional hospital was able to provide a full range of mental health services, including direct practice, consultation, and community development. However, the program had a waiting list for service and also lacked the resources to provide the intensive intervention requested by all the victims/survivors who came forward from this family. The local Social Services offices could not offer any assistance, since their mandate limited their involvement to children under the age of 16 years. The court-oriented victim services personnel could offer intervention to assist with court preparation only.

The family (i.e., sibling survivors), as a group, had approached all available and appropriate services within the local area but were unable to secure any intervention that would begin to address their crisis in any coordinated fashion. The magnitude of this crisis was such that no single agency was able to use a model of individual intervention and counseling to provide meaningful service to all of the siblings who came forward. In short, it was just too much for any one agency to manage on its own. Therefore, a combination of applicable community resources was the only viable option for an immediate and appropriate response.

SERVICE RESPONSE

To have any reasonable possibility of success, the service response had to address a number of essential issues discussed in the literature on intervention with victims/survivors of sexual abuse. These include:

1. Service facilitators had to be knowledgeable about the impact of abuse and able to effectively communicate to their client(s) that their experience and reactions to abuse were normal rather than an indication that they were crazy or mentally ill (Engel, 1989, p. 15).
2. Service facilitators had to be able to accept that their client(s) were telling the truth, no matter how brutal the abuse disclosed (Bass and Davis, 1988, pp. 345-346).
3. Service facilitators had to be sensitive to the issues of gender, and the preferences survivors may have to the gender of the counselor, which may be directly linked to the success of their intervention (Bass and Davis, 1988, p. 346).
4. Sexual abuse is an abuse of power. Counselors therefore had to be sensitive to the issues of power and power imbalance as they effect the therapeutic relationship (Lew, 1986, pp. 197-198).
5. A sense of safety had to be created and maintained, one in which anonymity is protected and confidentiality of both clinical content and records is secure, and the limits of confidentiality are made explicit (Health and Welfare Canada, 1991).

A team approach was developed, with a social worker recently hired by a small regional mental health service and a public health nurse who was native to the area and had worked in this capacity for almost five years. This was a functional composition of male and female cofacilitators with complementary clinical skills and common philosophies and beliefs (i.e., feminist approaches, holistic systems perspectives, etc.) about working with people.

The mental health social worker had a clinical background in the areas of individual and family therapy, including individual and group work experience in working with adult survivors of sexual abuse. The public health nurse had a clinical nursing background working with individuals and families with a focus on wellness and health promotion. Of equal importance, the public health nurse was well known in the community through her nursing practice and active involvement with the Bay St. George Women's Center. This level of community credibility enabled the family to feel safe enough to engage in an intervention process with a mental health service that was newly formed and staffed with personnel that were not from the local region. Additionally, the common areas of concern among the agencies and personnel within this rural region enhanced a networking process that facilitated the development of a quick and cooperative service response.

INTERVENTION

Intervention consisted of biweekly family/group sessions of two hours duration in an environment identified as safe by clients. The initial sessions focused upon fostering a safe environment in which all family members could openly articulate their relevant needs and voice their experiences as survivors, along with the associated affect. Each sibling had a need to speak of his/her experiences and to be heard; for many this was the first time. This intervention was unable to accommodate any individuals identified as perpetrators (i.e., criminal record). However, they did have the option of individual intervention from another clinician in the region. In retrospect, facilitators felt that providing the option of individual service to siblings identified as perpetrators (at least one was identified) was essential in securing the motivation of many of the siblings to engage in a group work process. Family loyalties were such that if some kind of intervention and assistance were not made available to all family members who requested it (including perpetrators) all service options would have been rejected on the principle that they were discriminatory or were abandoning a family member in need.

Contributing to the success of the process was the fact that both cofacilitators were explicit in outlining their experiences, backgrounds, and personal strengths and limitations, as well as the necessity of confidentiality of both clinical content and records and the limits of that confidentiality.

The eight siblings who engaged in counseling included seven females and one male, ranging in age from 22 to 44 years. Some shared a common community setting while others lived in areas by themselves. All but two of the younger sisters were married and had families of their own. Siblings had varied levels of education, positions of employment, and standards of living, ranging from university educated to functionally literate and from full or seasonal employment to being in receipt of social welfare.

The extent of physical and sexual abuse that each experienced also varied in magnitude and intensity. All experienced a childhood filled with extreme violence at the hands of their father. This physical and sexual abuse was either perpetrated upon themselves and/or had been witnessed happening to their sisters and brothers. The acts of violence ranged from indiscriminate beatings using bare hands or weapons (i.e., sticks, ropes, knives, firearms) to sexual assault, rape, prostitution of children, and forced sex with animals. Some maintained very vivid memories of many incidents from early childhood to the time they left home, while others recalled only partial memories or no memories at all.

All of the siblings were experiencing varying degrees of a number of psychological, emotional, and physical symptoms which the literature identifies as possible consequences of unresolved childhood sexual abuse. These included, but were not limited to: damage to self-esteem and self-image (i.e., feelings of worthlessness, feelings of being stupid/a failure/a loser, feelings of guilt, shame, helplessness, self-blame, and sabotaging success); relationship problems (i.e., difficulty trusting others, tendency to be involved with abusive people, intimacy problems, difficulty being assertive); emotional problems (i.e., unexpected and sometimes uncontrollable intense anger and rage, severe mood swings, dissociation, extreme fears, nightmares and night-terrors, posttrauma and flashbacks, substance abuse/addictions, and self-destructive behaviors); physical problems (i.e., somatic symptoms, tendency to be accident prone, physical illness); and problems in sexuality and sexual functioning (Mrazek and Mrazek, 1981, pp. 242-3; Engel, 1989, pp. 9-15).

The importance of positive, empowering client experiences during the commencement of therapy cannot be overemphasized since it lays the groundwork for future successful intervention. Upon successfully joining with the siblings of this family, the magnitude and intensity of the clinical issues could be assessed and approached from within the existing family system (Minuchin and Fishman, 1981). Only after the facilitators were accepted into the family system (i.e., structural family therapy approach of joining) was the process of intervention possible. Having achieved this, facilitators began the process of raising the siblings' awareness as to what actually constituted childhood sexual and physical abuse and its long-term impacts.

In fact, this education and awareness-raising process served as a catalyst for identifying and addressing the long-term issues that were most relevant for the siblings as individuals and as a family of survivors. The identification of relevant family issues was a source of common ground on which they could begin the practice of communicating with and supporting each other on a more functional level. Becoming aware of what constituted abuse and its effects afforded the opportunity for this family to understand that their feelings and affect to brutal childhood experiences were normal reactions, and not evidence that they were going collectively crazy. The facilitators stressed the importance of accepting all disclosures and graphic descriptions of brutal experiences as truthful. This validated the experiences of this family of survivors and fostered the development of a trusting relationship between the survivors and the facilitators.

The extensive use of the literature and self-help material developed by other survivors was pivotal in assisting this family to normalize their feelings and affect as normal reactions to childhood sexual and physical abuse. This included the use of literature and written materials (e.g., *The Courage to Heal*, Bass and Davis, 1988; *Adults Molested as Children: A Survivor's Manual for Women and Men*, Bear and Dimock, 1988; *Victims No Longer*, Lew, 1986; *Suffer Little Children*, O'Brien, 1991) and the access to similar materials on audio tape(s), as well as the use of video materials during group sessions (e.g., *To a Safer Place, Sandra's Garden*, and *The Boys of St. Vincent*).

In addition to normalizing their feelings and reactions to abuse, the use of these materials effectively reduced their sense of isolation (by showing that they are not alone as survivors) and offered them a sense of hope that healing was possible. In conjunction with the use of formal written and video-taped materials, the cofacilitators shared anecdotal material of the experiences of other survivors with whom they had worked. These stories of other survivors offered examples of practical coping strategies for daily living and for future healthy functioning (Laidlaw, Malmo, and Associates, 1990, pp. 3-4).

After several months of counseling, the issue of participation in the criminal proceedings against their aging father had to be addressed by the sisters and brothers within this group. With the trial of their father approximately two months away, and most group members subpoenaed to testify on behalf of the crown, group members identified the need to be informed of the legal system and the roles they would be required to play in this process. Group members had little knowledge of the legal system and this, in conjunction with the prospect of facing their father (their perpetrator) and his support people, evoked extreme anxiety, fear, and distress.

To address this, court preparation services were sought from the Victim's Services Branch of the Department of Justice. This was a relatively new service in the area at the time, with limited resources, normally providing court preparation services on an individual basis to victims of crime. Instead of having group members get involved in lengthy travel to avail themselves of this service on an individual basis, the service was offered in conjunction with regular sibling group sessions. This was achieved through consultation and consent of the family members in cooperation with the Victim Services Branch. In this manner, court preparation was enhanced because the issues of safety and support could be maintained within the integrity of the group setting. This method of service delivery was, in fact, beneficial to both consumers and service providers, as it was consumer friendly (adapted to meet client needs) and utilized less resources to deliver service.

OPPORTUNITY ARISING FROM A CRISIS

Shortly before the trial date, the perpetrator (i.e., the father of these siblings) was found dead in his place of residence. Although he was 70-years old and had a history of chronic medical problems, his death was unexpected. In light of the recent disclosures of incest and abuse, the criminal proceedings, and the general turmoil within the family, the father's death created a crisis of significant intensity. Just when the siblings in the group were preparing themselves to confront their perpetrator in court, they were faced with the crisis of his death. Not only were they unprepared for this occurrence, they were also faced with the emotional unbalancing of feeling directly or indirectly responsible for causing his death by their disclosures. In fact, many of their extended and immediate family blamed them for all of the recent disruption in the family, including their father's death.

Nowhere was the intensity of this crisis more evident than in the funeral home where the body was being waked. At the request of group members, both counselors attended the wake and facilitated the group process on site. Reframed, this method of service provision was no different from the counselors' plan to attend the trial where these sisters and brothers were to confront their perpetrator (Laidlaw, Malmo, and Associates, 1990, p. 5). Viewed from this perspective, this crisis was in fact an opportunity to address the issues of these survivors that would promote their process of healing. Again, this was another example of the benefits of service flexibility and adaptability in meeting the needs of clients.

PROGRESS IN PSYCHOSOCIAL FUNCTIONING

Within seven months of commencing group therapy all siblings had illustrated significant improvement in psychosocial functioning. This was evidenced by, but was not limited to, their ability to identify the impact incest and abuse has had upon their lives, their demonstrated ability to employ healthy strategies of coping with the impact of incest and abuse, their ability to appropriately assign the blame for the abuse to the abuser, their ability to identify the ways power and control had impacted their lives, and their ability to identify and demonstrate more functional family and interpersonal relationships.

The siblings demonstrated examples of progress in these areas throughout the process of therapy. However, nowhere was evidence of progress more apparent than in the direction they chose in confronting their issues of abuse at the funeral home during their father's wake. Their progress was highlighted at this time because they illustrated improved levels of functioning during a severe crisis when, in fact, they were also at most risk of regressing to previous dysfunctional methods of coping. The noted improvements in psychosocial functioning enhanced emotional, psychological, and physical wellness among members of this sibling group. This promotion of wellnes, in all likelihood, prevented the future necessity of more acute mental health intervention for some of these individuals. Closure was initiated by siblings and followed up by facilitators over a two-month period, during which time areas of progress and healing were debriefed. When resiliency in these areas appeared sound, as agreed upon by the group and the cofacilitators, the group formally concluded.

DISTINCTIVE ASPECTS OF GROUP WORK WITH SIBLING SURVIVORS

There were several aspects in this clinical approach of assisting victims/survivors of incest that significantly differentiate it from both more typical group work experiences and family therapy interventions. First of all, this was decidedly different from most group work interventions with victims/survivors in that all group members shared substantial aspects of their lives outside the group setting. In effect, each group session was a "snapshot" of a group process that was constantly ongoing in the daily lives of each of the siblings. This profoundly limited the capacity of invoking structured activities upon the group work process. Cofacilitators had structured activities and group exercises planned for each group session, but quite often the needs, as expressed by the group, superseded any planned activities. Often an issue or topic that was raised by one of the siblings strongly reflected those of others. Therefore, the issues that were raised, frequently during check-in, could require extensive time to properly debrief and problem-solve that was in many ways directly proportional to the shared nature of their lives.

Second, structure and planning in group work usually fosters a common therapeutic experience for all participants (Corey and Corey, 1987, pp. 10-11). This is true with regard to membership criteria, frequency and length of sessions, rules of conduct, and common issues among individuals (Shulman, 1984, pp. 186-90). Unlike other group work experiences involving multiple sexual abuse victims from a single offender (e.g., therapy group co-led by the mental health social worker for sexual abuse victims of a Roman Catholic priest), this group did not require a great deal of planned intervention strategies. They did, in fact, respond with less enthusiasm to planned intervention than to their own spontaneous issues. As a result, cofacilitators required a high degree of flexibility and adaptability to effectively meet the demands of this type of group process involving sibling survivors.

A third distinctive characteristic of this group, different from most other groups for incest and abuse survivors, was their capacity to organize and call emergency sessions on short notice when situations warranted. Although this occurred only twice during a nine-month period, both occasions were timely and necessary in addressing the individual and collective needs of group members. In fact, this characteristic is more typical of family therapy intervention.

A fourth aspect of this approach which differentiated it from most family therapy methods was that this intervention only involved siblings and no other family members. It was not initiated to address problem issues associated with children and adolescents (i.e., where the child is the identified patient), nor was intervention initiated to address marriage/couple difficulties within a family setting (Breunlin et al., 1988, p. 310; Broderick and Schrader, 1981).

LIMITATIONS OF APPROACH

The fact that marital issues could not be addressed within this group setting could be considered a limitation of the method. In fact, most if not all issues for partners of survivors (Davis, 1991) went unaddressed within the context of this intervention. A second limitation of this method of intervention was that it was not conducive to personal growth counseling. It is felt that the reasons for this limitation were the individual differences of the sibling members, especially in the areas of age, present life circumstances, educational levels, and gender. Counseling to address issues of personal growth with two of the siblings was approached on an individual basis after the group had concluded. It was the position of the facilitators, and of both siblings, that personal growth intervention (i.e., adult survivor's issues of childhood abuse and incest) was only possible after the individual and family crisis was addressed by the group work process.

A final component of this clinical experience which merits mention, but is not necessarily a limitation, is the enormous impact that this group process involving siblings had on the extended family. Only eight of the 18 siblings consented to and engaged in this group work intervention. The rest of the siblings and other extended family members (i.e., aunts, uncles, cousins) generally did not want any intervention services and many did not even acknowledge that disclosures of incest and physical abuse had occurred.

The result was a split in both the sibling and extended family systems. Many of the siblings who did not engage in the group work process, along with much of the extended family, disassociated themselves from the siblings who disclosed, and in many ways shunned them from future interaction. Though facilitators did address this consequence throughout the group work process, they were unable to adequately prepare the siblings involved for the intense reaction and resolve of the rest of the family. Facilitators feel that this result was, in many ways, inevitable and expect that a lengthy process of grieving at their loss of family will be a necessary aspect of their recovery.

REFERENCES

Bass, E. & Davis, L. (1988). *The Courage to Heal: A Guide for Women Survivors of Sexual Abuse*. Harper & Row, New York.

Bear, E. & Dimock, P. (1988). *Adults Molested as Children: A Survivor's Manual for Women and Men*. Safer Society Press, Orwell, VT.

Breunlin, D., Breunlin, C., Kearns, D. & Russell, W.(1988). A Review of the Literature on Family Therapy with Adolescents 1979-1987, *Journal of Adolescence*, Vol. 11, pp. 309-334.

Broderick, C. & Schrader, S. (1981). The History of Professional Marriage and Family Therapy, in Gurman, A. S. & Kniskern, D. P. (Eds.). *Handbook of Family Therapy*, (pp. 5-35). Brunner/Mazel, New York.

Corey, M. & Corey, G. (1987). *Groups: Process and Practice*. Brooks/Cole Publishing Company, Pacific Grove, CA.

Davis, Laura. (1991). *Allies in Healing*. Harper Collins, New York.

Engel, Beverley. (1989). *The Right to Innocence: Healing the Trauma of Child Sexual Abuse*. P. Tarcher. Los Angeles, CA.

Health and Welfare Canada. (1989). *Health Care Related to Abuse, Assault, Neglect and Family Violence Guidelines*.

Laidlaw, T. A., Malmo, C. & Associates. (1990). *Healing Voices: Feminist Approaches to Therapy with Women*. Jossey-Bass Publishers, San Francisco.

Lew, Mike. (1986). *Victims No Longer: Men Recovering from Incest and Other Child Sexual Abuse*. Harper and Row, New York.

Minuchin, S. & Fishman, H. C. (1981). *Family Therapy Techniques*. Harvard University Press, Cambridge, MA.

Mrazek, D. & Mrazek, P, (1981). Psychosocial Development Within the Family, in P. Mrazek & E. Kempe. *Sexually Abused Children and Their Families* (pp. 17-32). Pergamon Press, New York.

O'Brien, Dereck. (1991). *Suffer Little Children: An Autobiography of a Foster Child*. Breakwater Books, St. John's, NF.

Report of the Archdiocesan Commission of Inquiry into the Sexual Abuse of Children by Members of the Clergy. (1990). Winter Report, Archdiocese of St. John's.

Report of the Committee on Sexual Offenses Against Children and Youth. (1984). (Vol. 1), Badgley Report, Minister of Supply and Services.

Shulman, Lawrence. (1984). *The Skills of Helping: Individuals and Groups*. F. E. Peacock Publishers, Inc., Itasca, IL.

Chapter 16

A Community Center Model
for Current Urban Needs

John KixMiller
Helene Filion Onserud

During the past few years public policy discussions both in New York City and on a national level have focused increasing attention on the need for programs and community supports for young people. Especially in urban settings, the widespread social problems affecting adolescents (school failure, violence, pregnancy, drug addiction, crime, etc.) have drawn ever-growing concern and research from private foundations, the popular media, and the political arena. As an example, the Carnegie Council on Adolescent Development (1992) recently released a report on youth development and community programs titled *A Matter of Time: Risk and Opportunity in the Nonschool Hours*. After detailing the immense need for positive community involvement, adult guidance, and employment or preemployment opportunities for adolescents, the authors criticize current programs, describing them as "typically fragmented and uncoordinated . . . often address[ing] single problems . . . underfinanced," as suffering from "low morale" among staff, and tending to serve "more advantaged families." The authors state that:

> The time has come to change these conditions dramatically. Youth-serving agencies, government, and all sectors concerned about youth must join in an effort to expand opportunities for young adolescents when they are out of school, improve program quality and increase program intensity, and extend these activities particularly to young adolescents who live in low income often high-risk communities. (p. 12)

In general, there is agreement in the current literature on the need for youth development programs that provide for: (1) ways for youth to contribute positively to their larger community; (2) avenues toward work experience and employment; (3) ways for youth to be closely involved with each other and caring adults; and (4) extensive time commitments (more than a couple of hours a week) for youth, especially in "high-risk" communities. One major outcome of this intense policy discussion concerning youth development has been the Department of Youth Services funding of Beacon schools in New York City. The idea that public schools in each neighborhood should be open to youth and community service activities during the nonschool hours has to some extent become a practical reality that receives public funding.

However, it must be said that the nature of the professional tasks and form of program organization best suited to achieve youth development goals within Beacon schools and elsewhere remains in some dispute and confusion. A variety of models of youth development programs are offered from different sectors of the practice and research landscape (Cahill, 1993; Carnegie,1992; Sherraden, 1992), and it is clear that different models may be successful when concentrating on different tasks and goals. The most effective way to meet the needs of youth on a large scale and to spend public money for these services, however, remains a complex and controversial issue.

Michael Sherraden (1992), in his comparative study of youth programs in five different countries, writes that:

> Ideally, like many other western nations, the United States would develop a national perspective on youth professionals and establish educational standards defining a youth work training curriculum. However, in looking at other countries, the content of this curriculum remains largely undefined and there are many opinions about what it should be. This study does not give a clear picture of what youth workers should know and be able to do. And doing something distinctly well is, after all, the primary rationale for the existence of a profession. (pp. IX-X)

As Sherraden hints at the idea that a profession might be needed to give the field of youth development a solid anchor, it seems surprising that the profession of social work (and particularly social group work, with its rich tradition of working with youth) is not making a larger contribution to the theory and practice of youth development in the cities of the United States today. Grace Coyle, who was largely responsible for the recognition of social group work as a professional methodology within social work, wrote extensively about precisely this area of service which currently is being debated.

Coyle (1947, 1948, 1980) believed that community centers, settlement houses, and other forms of group work programs represented in fact a new institution that thoughtfully planned for the needs of a modern industrialized society, with particular emphasis on the socialization of children and youth. She stated:

> Obviously we, like all societies, rely largely on the family to perform many of the essential functions in the nurture of the younger generation. With our American traditions we have always put our faith in the school and the church as the major instrumentalities outside the home for these purposes. Within the past century, however, we have invented an additional institution. This new organ is our familiar set of organizations of, for, and by youth. (1948, p. 10)

Almost half a century later James Comer (who cochaired the interdisciplinary task force responsible for the recent report put forth by the Carnegie Council on Adolescent Development) prefaces *A Matter of Time* with ideas and descriptions echoing those put forth by Coyle. He writes that his experience in educational reform has led him to believe that "there was indeed a third leg to the triangle of human development. If family and school constitute two of these legs, as I believe they do, the third leg is surely those experiences that young people have in their neighborhoods and the larger community" (Carnegie Council, 1992, p. 18).

Comer goes on to describe some of the societal changes that have occurred since World War II and how these have affected youth development. He points to the current situation in which a postindustrial economy has made increasing demands on young people in terms of levels of education and training, while at the same time the family and community supports on which they could once rely have been eroded (pp. 18-19). Comer is convinced "of the importance of reinventing community." He goes on to say that, "This sense of place, of belonging, is a crucial building block for the healthy development of children and adolescents. And it is especially crucial for young people who are growing up in disadvantaged circumstances" (p. 19). Comer thinks that children and youth need not only to be socialized as a group, but to be integrated into a viable community as well. On this point Coyle also was eloquent. She believed that the socialization of youth should be integrated in a community building process and that involvement in community building should be one of the purposes of programs for youth (1948, p. 8).

As social group work became professionalized, its purpose evolved out of the roots it had in youth service organizations and settlement houses and stressed a vision of the individual and society as mutually responsible for each other. This brought about a dual commitment to the concept of personality development through group life on the one hand, and to democracy "through the development of the group toward socially desirable ends" (Phillips, 1957, p. 28) on the other.

But since Grace Coyle elaborated her ideas on the nature of an institution for the development of youth, very little prestige, status, financial rewards, or theoretical interest have been attached to this endeavor in the social sciences in this country, even within the profession of social work. As a result, the promising strides group workers made early on in this direction eventually were superseded by more rewarding ventures into clinical group work.

It would be outside the scope of this paper to give a full account of the causes underlying this change of orientation within the methodology, but a few important points can be made here. During the 1940s and 1950s, the professionalization of social group work was strongly influenced by its sister method, casework, which attracted attention to the therapeutic possibilities inherent in the new method. Eventually, this trend diverted attention from the early goals of social change, individual development, and community building. This is not to say that exploration of some of these aspects of group work was not continued. Emanuel Tropp, William Schwartz, (Roberts and Northen, 1976; Alissi, 1980) and William Rosenthal, among others, have done helpful work in elaborating this heritage during the last 30 years. But by and large the major trends today are towards treatment-oriented, problem-based group work.

As this change of orientation developed, the use of program activities, which had a central function in the early concept of the group and put the emphasis on "doing things together," was replaced by a "talk centered" modality, and over time practically disappeared. The use of expressiveness and creativity did come back to group work via psychology and psychiatry, but by then it was linked with therapy (Middleman, 1982, p. AM 48).[1]

Following these developments within the profession, more recent waves of conservatism have also eroded the base of support that organizations which were committed to the traditional social group work approach still had. Funding sources, often politically motivated, tend to control the nature of programs offered by social service agencies. This phenomenon has been reflected in the trend toward problem-based, categorical, and fragmented services, which even settlements and community centers have adopted over the community-building approach that was at one time central to these organizations using the social group work methodology.

As a result, the field of youth development does not mention social work as an available professional basis for program models and the training of youth development workers. But as the ideas which helped shape the social group work method (particularly the need for a new social institution for the development and socialization of youth, and the fact that teenagers as a group need to be integrated in society) are receiving increasing attention again, what can the tradition of social group work still offer to help deal with the urgent need for youth service programs today?

These authors believe that the social group work method, rooted as it is in social work ideas and principles, still presents us with a powerful response to the crisis we are facing at the present time.

Any model for a social institution must respond to needs clearly and commonly visible in typical neighborhoods. In general the youth development field focuses on children ages ten to 15, yet the literature continually stresses the need to integrate teens into the fabric of community life (Maas 1984). Recent studies (Carnegie, 1992; Sherraden, 1992) cite the isolation of teens on the margins of society as part of the problem hindering the maturation of teens into productive adults. Young teens are herded together in middle schools and are provided with few consistent links with younger children or adults. Most teens in general are unemployed and have little hope of becoming employed.

In making an assessment of social problems affecting teens, it is difficult to avoid an examination of the changing structure of family life in modern urban America. The startling rise of single-parent families and of families with two working parents over the past two decades has resulted in the absence of parents from the home during afterschool hours, and a diminishing capacity on the part of parents to spend time with and to structure the lives of their children (Fink, 1986; Miller and Mark, 1990). In addition, it is well documented that "the period from 1974 to the present marks the first time in the nation's history that children have been the poorest group in society" (United States, 1991, p. 29). Parents not only have less time for their children, they also have significantly less money.

The problems that disrupt teenagers' development have roots in their earlier years (Leventhal and Dawson, 1989). Children who are uninvolved with adults during much of their nonschool hours will find other role models to follow and copy. The most available role models on the streets, playgrounds, and unsupervised apartments in New York City are unemployed teens. The volatile mix of unsupervised children in daily association with unemployed teens has led to a subculture in urban settings whose values, including the use of weapons, alienation from school, and involvement in sexual activity, are often destructive of the kind of future most parents would prefer to envision for their children, and most young people would choose to have for themselves if given the chance. Yet parents cannot be encouraged to quit their jobs to spend more time with their children at home. Moreover, even those families with a parent at home often have trouble monitoring the nonschool social activities of older children and young teens.

Given this situation and what is known about youth development in urban settings in general, a coherent model for a community center that aims to address the developmental needs of teenagers has to integrate a community building process that also includes services for younger school-age children and for parents. These authors have participated in the development of such a model at the

Center for Family Life, a social work agency in Sunset Park, Brooklyn over the last decade.

A COMMUNITY CENTER MODEL

A community center involves the thoughtful creation of age-appropriate relationships and activities for all participants. It offers an environment where the developmental needs of various age groups are given a proper context in which to work out the issues related to these needs. The major purpose of a community center is to provide for the social life of its members in a way that represents the values of parents, the profession of social work, and the principles of political democracy and a multicultural society. To accomplish this a community center model must provide: (1) a holistic environment representing the various ages and developmental stages; (2) a variety of activities appropriate for peer groups of different age levels; and (3) a clear sense of adult authority representing professional and community values.

A Holistic Environment

The task of creating and maintaining a holistic environment representing the various ages and developmental stages of life is at the heart of any community center model. This task demands that the center function as an interrelated community rather than a series of fragments. It is a major psychological assumption of this professional approach that people need to experience a community of different age groups coming together, and that healthy individual identity is nourished by such an environment. Special events, including performing arts shows, multi-arts festivals, fashion shows, olympics, fairs, pot-luck dinners, and other community-wide events, have as their major purpose the opportunity of bringing different participants together and allowing groups to present themselves to a whole community. As the reader will see, other means can be found to bring groups together to a lesser degree on a daily basis.

The practical tasks of child care, and the professional and community values accompanying it, are among the most needed and best understood responsibilities in any community. The value of children and their well-being is a decisive experience in the life of virtually everyone. Therefore, using a school-age child care program as the integrative component for a community center provides a structure which allows for a wide range of age groups, activities, roles, and responsibilities to overlap and meet around a common purpose. It includes teens who volunteer their time working with children through a counselor-in-training program, and who then become committed to the success of that operation; young adults who have reached the level of maturity needed to become group leaders; and parents who naturally have a stake in the well-being of their children and of the community in which they live. A community center organized in this way supports the passages from childhood to adolescence and from adolescence to adulthood and makes itself highly visible to the whole community.

Activities for Peer Groups of Different Ages

The group provides a cohesive matrix, a step removed from the original family, to help work out the tasks of maturation. The skill of the worker goes into building a group that reflects the personal meaning of its members. Creative projects, athletics, social relations, a deepening relationship with authority figures, and community life are all pieces of personal meaning in the inner life of group members. An individual will react to these areas according to the state of his inner world. Tropp (1980) has coined the term "developmental group" to describe this form of group because the tasks of personality development are the group's basic agenda. From this point of view, a group member's conflicts with peers and authority can be seen as normal aspects of group process.

Children need to have a context in which they can play, or come together around activities as well as acquire and practice the skills that will allow them to gain mastery and feel competent in the accomplishment of a varety of tasks. They need to do this in the company of a group of peers with whom they can identify, form relationships, and interact freely. They also need role models and authority figures who can guide them, and with whom transference issues can be worked out.

In the context of a daily school-age child care program, it is important that children have an ongoing group. The structure of traditional after-school centers and day camps in which children are placed in groups according to age and sex with a stable leader is ideal for such a program.

Adolescents' developmental needs dictate a wider variety of options. In addition to the counselor-in-training program which provides the link for teens to the school-age child care program and to the rest of the community, there have to be other forms of peer groups in which young people can acquire skills and struggle with identity issues in various ways. Teens need to be able to choose a group based on their interests, level of skills, or their attraction to a group worker who can become a suitable role model for them. These can include sports teams, dance and acting groups, fashion groups, discussion groups focusing on important teen-age issues, youth councils, etc.

Parents should be given opportunities to participate in the community center as well. They can become members of a parents' advisory council, they can volunteer their time working with groups of children, or they can help plan and prepare for special events. They can also join activity groups. Generally, however, it seems to be difficult for parents to get involved in groups that focus on their needs as individuals. The pressures and demands of work and family life are great in an urban environment, and often do not give them the leisure to do something for themselves. Giving parents access to community center life through activities relating to their children, or through groups which they can join with them (such as intergenerational activity groups), provides a solution to the dilemma of parents' noninvolvement.

An established structure for youth leadership development and staff training must be a crucial feature of this model. This training can start as teens join the counselor-in-training program and intensify as they become young staff members, group leaders, or assistants. These young workers serve as role models and authority figures for large groups of children, and some of them for teens and parents as well. The psychological tensions of these relationships can easily be underestimated. Children can be struggling to resolve a variety of conflicts with a worker in a group setting that the worker him or herself is not necessarily able to handle. Emotional tasks concerning authority and other issues will call for levels of maturity in workers that have not yet been achieved. Therefore, workers must be provided with a setting in which to struggle with the steps they must take within themselves to handle their jobs. In this context, interpersonal relationships (as they relate to the program) are also part of the process. The staff group must present the model experience for all the other groups. Children cannot be asked to do activities or achieve levels of relating or understanding to which staff are not fully committed themselves.

Adult Authority Representing Professional and Community Values

A community center must present adult authority based on professional and community values through practical responsibilities and needed roles. The emotional and physical safety of children is a value that virtually everyone accepts, at least in theory. Therefore, the process of training teens as staff for a school-age child care program provides the clearest possible forum for presenting values and adult authority. Teens will accept very stringent training and a clearly defined code of behavior in order to provide safety and appropriate leadership to children. Moreover, within the overall dynamics of a community center, it is especially important that as children make the transition to adolescence they are offered the opportunity to work first on a volunteer and later, hopefully, on a paid basis. Children want to begin "helping" and psychologically need to see themselves on a path to productive adulthood.

It is not possible to combat the problems of urban youth subculture on a "just say no" basis. Adult authority must communicate a clear and convincing answer to the question "why?" The safety and appropriate leadership of children is an overwhelmingly effective answer. And even the future success of a basketball team or of a performing arts group will often suffice. On a broader level, the need to build a program or a safe community will begin to convince people of the importance of values and authority once they have had the chance to experience some of the benefits inherent in such an environment. But first, there must be real jobs, roles, and responsibilities to offer to people.

It is easy to criticize community center programs that make use of teen volunteers and staff from the point of view of professional child-care skills. It is certainly a major danger of this model that poor performance can be tolerated for the "good of teens," or that children can be used to give teens "responsibilities." Teens who enter a counselor-in-training program looking for a place to flirt and talk about the latest fight are not likely to have much attention to give to younger children. Yet, teens have major roles in the social-ization of their younger siblings all around the world and through-out history. To cast them as bad or incapable without giving them real responsibility in the life of their community is not an acceptable alternative. Adult staff must find ways–through supervision, staff meetings, and weekend retreats–to give teens the attention they need to do a good job. However, clearly not all teens are appropriate to work in child-care services. A variety of groups must be offered to meet the range of needs presented by adolescents. Various activi-ties such as sports, performing arts, tutoring, or creative arts all have productive goals and values appropriate to these purposes where adult authority has a well-understood, practical reason to exist.

Economics of the Model

One major purpose of community center programming is to support and strenghten neighborhood families. The ability of parents to survive and prosper economically is an essential factor in the health of any social structure. Moreover, legitimate economic incentives must exist within the grasp of adolescents to provide a bridge of transition from the world of childhood into the world of economically productive adulthood. Neighborhoods with scarce legitimate economic incentives and relatively few economically productive adults are necessarily fer-tile ground for producing the host of social ills associated with urban teens: crime, drug use, early pregnancy, and violence. From an eco-nomic point of view, what can this community center model offer to remedy this malaise?

Responsible and consistent school-age child care clearly helps par-ents go to school and hold jobs. Having to pick up their children at school every day at 3:00 p.m. is a major impediment to their holding a variety of available jobs. The cost of babysitting is often too high to make it worthwhile holding a job at all, especially when other issues are factored in, such as medical insurance and transportation. Helping parents to receive education and hold jobs is surely of primary eco-nomic importance to families and neighborhoods.

In addition, teens and young adults need local part-time jobs with a sense of mission. In effect, urban neighborhoods need an indigenous industry that can use the major labor force: unemployed teens and young adults who should be finishing high school and entering college. School-age child care and other community center programs provide the perfect vehicle for appropriate part-time jobs. These jobs are truly important and meaningful, and they are appreciated as such by the teenagers and young adults who hold them. Yet the jobs do not have to interfere with their going to school: they can actually be an incentive for them to stay in school. And the children need precisely these young people in leadership positions to provide them with role models they can accept and follow. The suitable labor force is exactly the people who need the jobs. This setting also provides the context for younger teenagers to receive a developmentally important preemployment experience as counselors-in-training. The cost of support services such as those offered through Project Youth, which could be very expensive in another context, are offset by the fact that the teenagers reinvest in the community center through their work.

CONCLUSION

Community center models which provide opportunities for youth involvement at a variety of levels are desperately needed as a response to the present urban crisis. This fact has been increasingly documented in much of the recent research on youth development. However, the unique feature of the model described in this chapter—based as it is on the traditional social group work methodology—is that in addition to offering solutions from preventive and economic perspectives, it provides a sound professional basis on which to conceptualize youth development, and for the training of youth development workers.

Forty-five years ago Grace Coyle thought that community centers and youth organizations similar to the model presented here provided a new social institution for the development of youth, and that the professionalization of social group work established a theoretical framework for this purpose. In the intervening years, however, very little has been done in social work to build on these foundations, either in theory or in practice. It is these authors' belief, nonetheless, that the need remains for a social institution which would integrate youth development in a community-building process, and that social group work is still in the best position to provide a professional foundation for it.

If social group work is to be involved in professionalizing youth development, however, it must foster the type of professional leadership described in this model. It must also attract students in social work schools who are representative of the young people from various ethnic and cultural groups residing in urban settings. These are the people who are most needed as administrators and other professionals in present-day urban community centers, because they are the most suitable role models and because they are particularly aware of the needs of young people growing up in urban neighborhoods. The involvement of social work schools in providing training for this type of service in itself would go a long way in attracting young people such as the ones involved in the model described above, since it would present them with a professional avenue to continue the training they already started and to build on the commitment they have to this type of work.

The profession of social work has another very important role to play in this endeavor. Its strength as a recognized and important player in the field of social services is needed to advocate for this type of model with policymakers and funding sources, and to take a stand against the present trend toward categorical funding and fragmented services for youth.

NOTE

1. The Midleman book, *The Non-Verbal Method in Working with Groups*, was reissued in 1982 by Practitioner's Press. Additional material was added and those pages are designated AM.

REFERENCES

Alissi, Albert S. (Ed.). (1980). *Perspectives on Social Group Work Practice.* New York: Free Press.
Cahill, Michele. (1993). *Creating a Network of After-School Education Programs: A Concept Paper.* New York: Youth Development Institute Fund for the City of New York.

Carnegie Council on Adolescent Development. (1992). *A Matter of Time: Risk and Opportunity in the Nonschool Hours.* Report of the Task Force on Youth Development and Community programs. New York: Carnegie Corporation.

Coyle, Grace L. (1947). *Group Experience and Democratic Values.* New York: Woman's Press.

————. 1948. *Group Work with American Youth.* New York: Harper.

————. 1980. "Some Basic Assumptions about Social Group Work." *Perspectives on Social Group Work Practice.* (Ed.) Albert Alissi. New York: Free Press.

Fink, Dale B. (1986). *Latchkey Children and School Age Child Care: A Background Briefing.* Wellesley: Wellesley College Center for Research on Women.

Leventhal, Bennett, and Kenneth Dawson. (1989). "Middle Childhood: Normality as Integration and Interaction." *Normality and the Life Cycle.* (Eds.) Daniel Offer and Melvin Sabshin. New York: Basic.

Maas, Henry. (1984). "Reciprocity and Caring Community." *People and Context: Social Development from Birth to Old Age.* Englewood Cliffs, NJ: Prentice Hall.

Middleman, Ruth R. (1982). *The Non-Verbal Method in Working with Groups.* Hebron: Practitioners.

Miller, Beth M., and Fern Marx. (1990). "Afterschool Arrangements in Middle Childhood: A Review of the Literature." Action Research Paper 2. Wellesley: Wellesley College Center for Research on Women.

Phillips, Helen U. (1957). *Essentials of Social Group Work Skill.* New York: Association.

Roberts, Robert W., and Helen Northen. (Eds.). (1976). *Theories of Social Work with Groups.* New York: Columbia UP.

Sherraden, Michael. (1992). *Community-Based Youth Services in International Perspective.* Washington: Carnegie Council on Adolescent Development and William T. Grant Foundation Commission on Work, Family and Citizenship.

Tropp, Emanuel. (1976). "A Developmental Theory." *Theories of Social Work with Groups.* (Eds.) Robert W. Roberts and Helen Northen. New York: Columbia UP.

————. (1980). "A Humanistic View of Social Group Work: Worker and Members on a Common Level." *Perspectives on Social Group Work Practice.* (Ed.) Albert Alissi. New York: Free Press.

United States. National Commission on Children. (1991). [Final Report] *Beyond Rhetoric, A New American Agenda for Families.* Washington: GPO.

Chapter 17

What Works in the Treatment of MICA Clients? A Journey Through the Evolution of an Outpatient MICA Program

Elizabeth A. Lewis

The purpose of this chapter is to acquaint the reader with information that will be of value in setting up a MICA program. Included is a brief history, current policy, a review of the current literature, and a description of the evolution of an outpatient program from its inception to its present form.

HISTORY

The deinstitutionalization and noninstitutionalization movements that began in the 1950s presented communities across the nation with many unexpected problems. One of these was the emergence of a large subgroup of severely and persistently mentally ill people, the mentally ill chemical abuser (MICA).

In 1955 the Joint Commission on Mental Illness and Health published a report that recommended developing community mental health centers and decreasing the size of mental hospitals. Synchronistically, the 1950s brought with them the increased use of neuroleptic medications for the mentally ill. This allowed severely mentally ill persons to have a degree of control over their symptoms and enabled them to live in communities rather than in inpatient units in psychiatric hospitals. The basic precept of deinstitutionalization was a commitment to provide the consumers of mental health services with adequate care in the least restrictive environment possible. The Community Mental Health Act of the 1960s placed a greater emphasis on treating the mentally ill within the communities. "In the early years after the Act, most of those seen were older, with long histories of institutionalization. During the past two decades, community mental health centers have seen an increasing number of younger adults, without the long experiences of hospitalization . . . " (Aliesan and Firth, 1990, p. 25). Substance abuse is a primary factor distinguishing the younger generations of psychiatric patients from their older counterparts. (Bauer, 1987, p. 1).

Of all chronically mentally ill adults, ages 18 to 40, literature estimates indicate that 20 percent to 80 percent have substance abuse problems. The discrepancy in research outcomes is a result of (1) the criteria used for diagnosis of both disorders and (2) the observation that "alcoholism (and drug use) can mask, mimic, precipitate or coexist with the gamut of psychiatric disorders" (Attia, 1988, p. 53). This makes diagnosis, and hence prevalence, extremely difficult to ascertain. However, even the most conservative figures demonstrate that there is an inordinately high number of substance abusers among the severely mentally ill compared to the general population.

Why do such a high percentage of mentally ill people abuse substances? There are several explanations offered in the literature. Communities are not adequately set up to care for the unique problems of the mentally ill. There exists a lack of tolerance for this population, many of whom look eccentric, are unable to hold down jobs, and at times end up homeless or otherwise displaced. A percentage of MICA clients can be found in jails. "Associated with substance abuse was a larger number of law violations mostly while intoxicated or stealing to finance drug purchases . . . " (Bauer, 1987, p. 3). They are engaged in a downward social drift into living settings in poor urban areas in which drug use and purveyance are common" (Drake, McLaughlin, Pepper, and Minkoff, 1991, p. 5). Intoxication generally has the effect of easing social situations, relieving boredom, assuaging anxiety and auditory hallucinations, and other symptoms of mental illness. It is a very "normal" way to socialize and receive acceptance from peers. In the long run, howev-

er, the substances tend to exacerbate psychiatric symptoms and lead
to a high rate of hospital recidivism and other social problems for the
mentally ill chemical abuser (Ryglewicz, 1989, ch. 4).

POLICY

Although the commission on mental health identified the plight of
the mentally ill chemical abuser in 1977, the service system is still
floundering in its ability to serve these people in a comprehensive
and relevant fashion. The reasons for this are numerous. The literature has cited the lack of willingness and ability of professionals to
make an accurate diagnosis of a dual disorder as being the single
most problematic issue interfering with adequate treatment delivery.
Funding streams in many states remain separate for mental health,
alcoholism, and substance abuse. Turf becomes a complicated issue
when MICA services are involved. "Programs cannot easily combine to become more responsive to the needs of mentally ill substance abusers when dollars remain separately targeted and tracked"
(Thacker and Tremaine, 1989, p. 1047). Schools do not provide
training in treating this population, so social workers and nurses,
alcohol and drug counselors and other front-line workers are not
prepared to deal with the special problems of MICA clients. Funding
has been scarce for new projects due to the state of and priorities of
the economy, leaving a paucity of research on MICA treatment and,
hence, few models for implementation of treatment programs.

Historically MICA clients have either been treated for their mental health problems in inpatient or outpatient mental health facilities, or have been treated for their substance abuse disorders in
detoxification and rehabilitation centers or outpatient substance
abuse treatment clinics. In traditional mental health philosophy,
substance abuse was viewed as "a symptom of underlying pathology or conflicts, and their failure to address it in direct and practical
terms led to great mistrust on the part of the recovering community" (Zweben and Smith, 1989, p. 221). By the same token, substance abuse treatment programs came into being and identified that
in many cases of recovering individuals, once recovery was under-
way, what had appeared as pathology was eliminated. "This led to
an under-recognition of pre-existing psychopathology, often to the

detriment of recovering patients who were often unable to establish or consolidate abstinence without having their other problems addressed" (Zweben and Smith, 1989, p. 221).

> This separation of treatment services is due, in part, to having different and sometimes conflicting treatment philosophies, theories, models, training and expectations. These in turn sometimes create differences in diagnosis, treatment goals, plans and strategies, measures of successes, appropriateness of pharmacotherapies; policies and procedures, length of treatment and outcome expectations. (Aliesan and Firth, 1990, p. 25).

TRADITIONAL SUBSTANCE ABUSE TREATMENT

Substance abuse treatment is traditionally offered using a group modality where motivation for recovery must be high, and abstinence agreed to. Strong confrontation by peers and group leaders is the method used to break through denial (Sciacca, 1987, p. 5). Staff often consists of people who are themselves in recovery and a high level of self-disclosure is required. The phases of treatment include:

1. *Acute stabilization:* This generally takes place in detoxification units where average length of inpatient stay is three to seven days. During this time, medications to assist with the detoxification may be administered by an MD. Staff will attempt to engage the patient in a rehabilitation program.
2. *Rehabilitation:* The beginning of rehabilitation can take place in either an inpatient program or an outpatient clinic. Groups are the mode of treatment and strong confrontation is integral to breaking down resistances and denial. Rehabilitation programs run from two weeks to two years, the most common lasting from four to six weeks.
3. *Ongoing rehabilitation and maintenance:* After participating in a rehabilitation program the consumer of substance abuse services generally engages in a self-help 12-step program. (Rehabilitation is not a prerequisite for attendance in 12-step programs.) In many communities 12-step groups are available on a seven-day-a-week basis. Attendance at these meetings is

voluntary and participants involve themselves as often and for as long as they feel is indicated to maintain abstinence, learn coping, and use the meetings for a support system.

Motivation for treatment and agreeing to abstinence are conditions of rehabilitation throughout each step of substance abuse treatment programs (Sciacca, 1991, p. 72). Urine screenings, breathalizing, and blood screenings are an important part of most substance abuse programs. If relapse occurs, the service consumer can start from detoxification, if necessary, or can go back into a rehabilitation program if physical dependence on the substance is not problematic.

Psychoactive medications are strongly discouraged as evidenced by the adage "a drug is a drug" (Attia, 1988, p. 60). This is an ideology that is changing as the field of substance abuse is beginning to recognize the plight of members who are unable to function well without prescribed psychotropic medications. AA and NA have the reputation for being antimedication (Zweben and Smith, 1989, p. 226). Twelve-step literature does not take this stance, yet many meetings still discourage the use of these medications.

Traditional mental health treatment includes:

1. *Acute stabilization:* This includes the stabilization of a multitude of psychiatric symptoms in inpatient psychiatric units in either psychiatric hospitals or on psychiatric units of general hospitals. Hospitalization can last from a brief visit in an emergency room to several years. The psychiatric condition is stabilized by the use of medications, low environmental stimulation, and structuring of time. When housing, benefits, and a follow-up program are in place, the patient is discharged.

2. *Rehabilitation and maintenance:* This takes place in either a day-treatment facility or in an outpatient mental health clinic. Day treatment often requires the consumer to be present several days per week. The client is scheduled with various activities throughout each day, including groups, individual therapies, social skills training, psychoeducation, socialization, case management, and medication services. An outpatient clinic will provide similar services; however, the consumer does not have a daily schedule at the clinic, rather, he or she comes in on a regular basis for a group or individual therapy session. Treat-

ment is offered on a needs basis. Many participants in outpatient clinic services have jobs or other activities that structure their time.

3. *Continuing Support Service (CSS):* Programs are set up with the understanding that even when a consumer has achieved some management of his/her symptoms, there remains a strong potential for relapse. The need for services may last for many years and perhaps for life.

THE MICA CLIENT DEFINED

MICA clients have been identified as being difficult to engage in services. They are notorious for having a high hospital recidivism rate whether treated in substance abuse services or mental health services. Across the board they have been looked upon as being treatment resistant. "Young adults (psychiatric patients) with ongoing substance abuse had an annual rate of psychiatric hospitalization that was over two and one-half times the rate for comparison groups where substance abuse was less" (Bauer, 1987, p. 3).

A comparison between MICA clients and mental health consumers who do not use substances show that MICA clients are younger and more often male, and they are less able to manage their lives in the community, i.e., eating regular meals, procuring adequate finances, living in stable housing, and engaging in regular activities. They show greater hostility, suicidality, and poorer medication compliance. Their hospital recidivism rate is higher (Drake and Wallach, 1989, p. 1041). MICA clients report greater levels of physical ills, depression, anxiety, obsessive-compulsiveness, paranoia, and psychotic symptoms. They also reported greater overall distress than non-substance abusing clients (Carey, Carey, and Meisler, 1991, p. 136).

Would MICA clients maintain the same profile of being "treatment resistant" if they were offered MICA specific treatment that addressed their concomitant illnesses? In a study done by Ries and Ellingson (1990), of 48 directors of inpatient psychiatric centers, 10 percent offered substance abuse treatment on their psychiatric units (p. 1230). "Over a third of patients in general psychiatric settings and half or more of those in settings that provide more intensive treatment, . . . have problems substantially affected by substance abuse or dependence" (Drake, McLaughlin, Pepper, and Minkoff, 1991, p. 3). In another study the

> major finding was that patients who traditionally are under-served by the service delivery system, participated in and responded favorably to treatment designed to meet their specific needs. . . . The patient's alcohol and other drug use diminished. Symptoms of mental disorder stabilized and remained controlled. Hospitalization rates declined. (Hanson, Kramer, and Gross 1990, p. 113-14)

Special MICA Concerns

Several issues that are relevant to understanding the needs of MICA consumers have been prevalent in the literature. One is the notion of involving the family in the treatment process. Several programs support the idea that consumers of MICA services benefit from family members having the opportunity to learn about mental illness and substance abuse and explore coping skills (Test, 1981; Reilly, 1987; Osher and Kofoed, 1989). Family therapy is offered in individual sessions or in multiple family groups. Family education is especially helpful because families learn about the illness in a blame free environment and feel more receptive to trying new approaches with their relatives.

Whenever the development of a MICA program is being considered, the role of drug screening or toxicology tests being built into the program should be well thought out. Carey (1989) states that having this available supports the participant in sobriety and helps to break through denial (p. 5).

Another important concept to consider when working with MICA clients is how to measure success. In traditional substance abuse treatment, total abstinence and reintegration into mainstream society are the measures of success. In mental health treatment the absence of symptoms of the mental illness and a degree of reintegration into society may signify success to the clinician. In MICA treatment, success may be recognized by acknowledging small increments of increased social interaction or a decrease in the use of substances, a decrease in the number of psychiatric hospitalizations, or some stabilization of symptoms of either disorder (Aliesan, 1990, p. 28).

Medication is an issue that continually needs to be addressed and supported. Often MICA clients are going through an investigation with their prescribing psychiatrist to find the most beneficial combination of medications that have the fewest or least bothersome side effects. Clients are often uncomfortable and feel as if they are being used for experimentation. Side effects can be very troublesome, leading to noncompliance with medications. Why a prescribed drug and not a street drug? This is a commonly asked question. Many MICA clients have been through programs that undermine the use of prescribed psychoactive medications. They have experienced rejection as a result of using these medicines. Reeducating the MICA consumer about medications and assisting them with tolerating medication trials are essential elements in increasing compliance with the search for the best medication regimen.

It is essential for the MICA client to have the opportunity to explore the relationship between his/her drug and alcohol use and psychiatric symptoms. "Group leaders and members assist individuals to gain insight into the dynamics and patterns of the use of the substances . . . " (Sciacca, 1987, p. 5).

Many MICA clients, though they may not seem to use substances to excess, have "an exquisite sensitivity" to these substances.

> There were many whose use of drugs or alcohol would not be regarded as excessive or problematic by most standards. However, this use appeared to exacerbate their psychiatric symptoms, decrease the effectiveness of chemotherapy, and thus directly or indirectly precipitate admissions to the hospital. (McKelvy, Kane, and Kellison, 1987, p. 23)

Integrated Treatment Models

It is interesting to note that over the past four years the literature has moved on from discussing the problems inherent in identification of MICAs and proposing the inclusion of interdisciplinary team members in various drug, alcohol, and mental health-based programs to actual proposals for simultaneous treatment of both disorders within the variety of treatment settings.

In the past several years some different models of integrated treatment have been considered and operationalized. Several themes in MICA treatment have emerged since the literature became focused on models of treatment:

1. There is a need for phase specific treatment. MICA clients come from a full spectrum of readiness for treatment, from crisis stabilization to actively working on recovery issues. Rehabilitation is a lengthy process even after long periods of abstinence from substances (Lehman, Myers, and Corty, 1989; Kaufman, 1989; Attia, 1988; Osher and Kofoed, 1989; Minkof, 1989).

2. Both illnesses need to be addressed simultaneously, either through a hybridized program or through a program that utilizes a case manager to coordinate care across agencies (Ridgley, Goldman, and Willenbring, 1990; Hanson, Kramer, and Grass, 1990; Lehman, Myers, and Corty, 1989).

3. Maintenance and rehabilitation are long processes that take years to accomplish (Lehman, Myers and Corty, 1989; Minkoff, 1989).

4. Medication is an issue that needs to be sensitively addressed throughout treatment (Zweben and Smith, 1989; Osher and Kofoed, 1989.)

5. Education about the illnesses is a necessary component of treatment (Sciacca, 1987; Flowers and Booraem, 1991; McKelvy, Kane, and Kellison, 1987; Attia, 1988; Osher and Kofoed, 1989).

6. The use of groups is paramount to educating, to the relearning of social skills and to the development of a social support system (Flowers and Booraem, 1991; McKelvey, Kane, and Kellison, 1987; Osher and Kofoed, 1989).

7. Groups should be heterogeneous regarding diagnoses and substances used and homogenous regarding level of functioning (Aliesan and Firth, 1990; Flowers and Booraem, 1991; Kaufman, 1989).

8. Abstinence is not necessarily a prerequisite for involvement in a MICA program although working toward abstinence will

be an eventual goal of treatment (McKelvy, Kane, and Kellison, 1987; Osher and Kofoed, 1989.)

9. A soft approach to relapse and "confrontation" is utilized, rather than the rigid confrontational approach used in substance abuse treatment programs (Hanson, Kramer, and Grass,1990; Sciacca, 1987; McKelvy, Kane, and Kellison, 1987; Osher and Kofoed, 1989).

10. MICA treatment will be part of a comprehensive program that offers support in areas such as employment, education, housing, and health care (Pepper and Ryglewicz, 1984; Test, 1981; Osher and Kofoed, 1989).

11. Although controversial, most treatment protocols include attendance at self-help groups. Several authors advocate for clients being taught to use the groups in a constructive way. Others suggest that MICA staff help clients choose meetings that are more tolerant of MICA members (Zweben and Smith, 1989; McKelvey, Kane, and Kellison, 1987; Attia, 1988; Reis and Ellingson, 1990; Minkoff, 1989). Some ideas for starting MICA-tailored self-help groups will be discussed further in this chapter.

Several authors have drawn a strong parallel between the concepts in treatment of the two disorders of major mental illness and substance abuse. Minkoff (1989) has proposed a treatment model based on these parallels. He states, "In each model the illness has a complex, multifactorial etiology, in which a hereditary or congenital biologic predisposition interacts with psychosocial stressors to result in the emergence of symptoms." He goes on to state that denial is paramount in each of the illnesses and that treatment needs to be primarily focused on this in the beginning phases. Addiction and psychosis are both characterized by a loss of control over some aspects of thinking and behaving (p. 1032). Understanding that a commonality exists between these two treatment models allows us to begin looking at ways to merge the separate philosophies into a unified treatment protocol. This notion sets the groundwork for formulating integrated, hybrid programs for the dually diagnosed.

THE EVOLUTION OF A MICA PROGRAM

This MICA program was conceived and birthed in a rural New York state outpatient mental health clinic in early 1988. The Continuing Support Services (CSS) unit had been in existence since the mid-1970s, offering services to the severely and persistently mentally ill. There were service consumers from this population who used alcohol or drugs from the beginning of the CSS program, yet the problem was not made overt until more than a decade later.

Stage I: Recognition of the Problem (Conception)

Clients at the CSS unit were offered weekly sessions of psychotherapy and case management services appropriate to someone who had marginal community living skills. Everyone knew David and Keith used cocaine and pot along with alcohol and their prescribed medications. No one gave this problem a name or gave much thought to how the coexistence of these two problems (mental illness and substance abuse) might impact on treatment outcomes. Some clients were encouraged to go to AA or NA meetings. A few clients were referred to substance abuse programs. A very few of those referred had positive results from the experience. Others could not make use of the style of treatment offered, due to the rigid rules and heavy confrontation. Far more CSS consumers were refused entry into substance abuse rehabilitation programs because of their mental illness or because they took psychotropic medications. Treatment in the CSS unit was focused on interpersonal problems, and case management issues such as housing, benefits, employment, daily structure, and the like. Substance abuse issues were largely overlooked.

In January 1988 a substance abuse program within the county system closed down because of lack of funding. Staff members from that program were assimilated into other county mental health units. A member of the alcohol team was assigned to the CSS unit. As this new staff member was intaking clients into the unit, she became acutely aware of the number of CSS clients who had concurrent substance abuse problems. This was the first time that dually diagnosed clients were identified as a subpopulation of CSS recipients. This new staff member requested permission to start a

MICA group, and it was granted. Basically this group was alcohol education, simplified and concretized, for chronically mentally ill people. This was not what the literature would consider an integrated approach, but more like concomitant services that were provided separately from each other.

Referrals for the group were made by CSS staff in response to a memo distributed by the organizing staff member. The group met for the first time at the end of April, with two group members and one staff member. The group was ongoing and new members came as they were referred. Criteria for the program included being dually diagnosed and being able to tolerate groups. Membership grew steadily. In six months there were 26 clients on the roster. The average attendance at a group was five members. After two months the original MICA group facilitator was joined in coleadership by the head of another substance abuse program in the county system. This staff member, as the first, did not have experience with the mentally ill. It is reported that he "spoke over the heads" of the group members. It was observed that the clients responded to his lectures with blank stares. He was apparently oblivious to his effect on the group members. In this embryonic stage of MICA program development it can easily be identified, as the literature states, how:

1. mental health professionals tended to be unaware of substance abuse as a significant problem, and
2. traditional substance abuse treatment (as administered by the second group facilitator) was not suited to severely mentally ill people.

Stage II: The Emergence of Integrated Treatment

In May 1989 funding for the substance abuse program was reinstated and the alcohol unit staff member left the MICA group to return to the alcohol program. A CSS staff member with a background in geriatric day programming was beginning work on the unit. In his interview for the job he requested groupwork and was put in charge of the MICA group. He had no formal experience with substance abusers, but had been involved in a day-treatment program for chronically mentally ill people. He was told to "show videos" on substance abuse. Members were at varied levels of functioning and the range of diagnoses covered the gamut of major mental illnesses and substance abuse. Attendance was sporadic and group cohesion was not thought of as an issue. The purpose of the group was to give information about how drugs and alcohol affect the user. When the county's supply of substance abuse videos was exhausted, they were shown again. When it seemed that reshowing the videos another time was overdoing it, the facilitator went to the local rural library to find new material.

During this stage of the MICA program there were times when one or two members would show up for group. After several months of videos, this new leader worked to give the program some variety. He had staff from alcohol and drug programs come in to talk to the group. The groups were 45 minutes long with a break in the middle. This facilitator stated that "people in the agency didn't think MICA clients were capable of much." When he tells this he chuckles at what is obviously an understatement. During his tenure as MICA group facilitator, this staff member lengthened the groups to an hour and a quarter with a break. It was felt that more women might join the group if this male facilitator had a female coleader. The person selected for this position came from a substance abuse background. The groups continued with approximately the same profile as before. The joining of a mental health worker with a substance abuse worker to facilitate the same MICA group was a significant event in the evolution of the program. This happened at the same time that CSS unit staff had become increasingly aware that MICA clients were not getting the treatment they needed from the agency.

Stage III: Birth of a Multiphase MICA Program

While these two staff members were coleading the MICA group, awareness of MICA issues was becoming more overt across the nation. The unit leader of CSS petitioned the agency for a staff position to develop a program. In late 1989 a social worker with substance abuse experience and a strong group work background was hired as the MICA program coordinator.

Her first clinical task was to provide supervision to both facilitators of the existing MICA group. She notes that there were basic conflicts between these two workers that stemmed from their diverse clinical orientations. The mental health worker was concerned about "coming on too strong with the clients," and the substance abuse worker felt that the approach was "too lax," and she wanted more confrontation between members. This dichotomy in approaches to early MICA treatment is frequently identified in the literature of the late 1980s. The program coordinator helped these group leaders negotiate a compromise in their approaches to the MICA group. Other major first tasks included providing in-service education for the MICA staff and negotiating a functioning, effective MICA program with few resources.

Though the coordinator of the new program wondered at times if she was "in over her head," she came up with a comprehensive plan for MICA services using available staff and not knowing where the funding was going to come from. The agency was supportive of new projects and administration told her to go ahead with the plans for the program, stating funding would be worked out in time. MICA treatment was becoming a major concern of the Office of Mental Health and anticipating funding for such a program was a small risk on the part of the agency.

After a year and a half of one strictly educational group that was ongoing and heterogeneous in terms of diagnoses and level of functioning, the new program director presented a plan for a full MICA program. This plan was based on a needs assessment indicating that approximately 44 percent of the clients enrolled in the Continuing Support Services unit of the agency had concomitant substance abuse problems. It should be noted that because it was mental health professionals submitting the forms for the needs assessment, it is likely that 44 percent is a conservative estimate (Thacker and Tremaine, 1989, p. 1046).

The original proposal was based on reviewing successful MICA programs that were in operation. The basic concepts adapted from these programs are listed in the original proposal. They are:

1. Both disorders are treated simultaneously; one diagnosis is not considered more primary than the other. (This had been a topic exhausted in the literature up to this time. There was a major emphasis on determining which diagnosis was primary in or-

der to be able to design a treatment plan before hybrid programs were available.)

2. Abstinence is expected as a goal and required while in attendance. (Abstinence as a goal rather than a prerequisite for admission into the program is a MICA concept as differentiated from a commitment to abstinence in substance abuse treatment.)

3. A drug-free environment is maintained providing new social supports to increase the motivation for abstinence. (This is also true in traditional substance abuse treatment.)

4. Psychoeducation on substance abuse and mental illness is emphasized. (In the existing group, psychoeducation about mental illness was not considered. This is an example of concomitant treatment that is not integrated.)

5. Relaxation skills and recreational activities reinforce the potential to enjoy life without chemicals.

6. Continuity of care exists with liaisons to inpatient, residential, and vocational programs. (These are services that already exist within the CSS care structure. All clients will be connected with these services through the larger CSS unit if admitted into the MICA program.)

7. Outreach to difficult, resistant clients. (This was an important concern; however, with a few minor exceptions, the agency was not able to afford this service.)

The program started in September 1990 with four part-time staff and the full-time coordinator. The proposal was based on a group-work model. All groups were co-led by a female and male facilitator. There were three reasons for this decision:

1. MICA clients can become easily overwhelmed or symptomatic. If this happened to a member, one of the facilitators could tend to the problem while the other facilitator could keep the group going.

2. A facilitator of each gender would ensure comfort for those who had issues with one gender. Having two facilitators would encourage role modeling within the group.

3. There was the consideration that "two heads are better than

one," especially when working with a population where the problems are so diverse and complex.

A "first-step" group was proposed for MICA clients who were either not yet committed to abstinence, or were psychiatrically unstable. This group met once a week for 50 minutes. The focus of this group was on psychoeducation about both illnesses and how members experienced each illness and their interactions. Verbal exchanges between clients were encouraged by the facilitators, and keeping discussions concrete in nature was emphasized. An NA meeting, held at the clinic, was offered to the first-step group. The NA meeting was chaired by an NA member who was tolerant of MICA issues including the use of prescribed psychotropic medications. This meeting was an hour long and met directly after the first-step group.

The other level of MICA treatment offered was the "full program." This was offered to clients who had a commitment to abstinence. The "full program" was scheduled for two hours, two days per week. On the first day there were two groups back to back, both lasting 50 minutes. The first group was called Substance Abuse Recovery Group, renamed by a group member "SARG." The purpose of this group was to provide education that would support the member in abstinence. This group was followed by the "GYST" group. Although, formally the acronym stood for "Get Your Stuff Together," the members renamed it "Get Your Shit Together." The purpose of this group was to provide an interactive, dynamic experience that would cover a range of topics such as health, nutrition, exercise, women's and men's issues, relaxation, and creative expression. On the second day, a Sobriety Skills group offered exploration of topics such as relapse prevention and 12-step preparation. The focus was on helping the client maintain sobriety. After the Sobriety Skills group, these clients were strongly encouraged to attend the MICA NA group along with the first-step members.

One more group was offered once a month for a group of the full-program members who had achieved three months or more of abstinence. This was the only group that was not co-led. Its purpose was to address the recovery issues of both mental illness and substance abuse in a group process format.

One thing all MICA staff members have learned through the past few years of facilitating MICA groups and promoting MICA treatment is that flexibility and open-mindedness are key elements to a surviving/successful program. The program began as proposed, and many elements of the original proposal are still in effect today. However, many elements have changed as MICA needs at the different levels of treatment have been identified and as members have grown and demanded more flexibility in their treatment.

Stage IV: Growth and Further Evolution

As time went on it became evident that another group was emerging. These were the MICA clients who were steadfast in their commitment to use their substance and yet willing to engage in an educational group. The first step group had advanced beyond this stage to a group that shared its time equally between didactic programming and group process. Members had become committed to abstinence, yet most still either did not have the stability to join the "full program" groups or were too attached to their own group to want to "advance" to the next level of treatment. In response to this dilemma, a new group was started in January 1992. The "drop-in group" was originally set up as a waiting list group from which members would eventually be integrated into either the first-step or full-program groups. As this group evolved it became evident that there were a number of participants who would be in this level of treatment and not necessarily progress to first-step. Attendance in the drop-in group was encouraged, but if members could not come, this was tolerated. In other levels of treatment, the cohesion of the group was considered as important to the group as the content. The drop-in group is the most didactic of all the groups. There is a time set aside for interaction, but no member is pushed to contribute. What started out as a waiting list group now has 27 members, some of whom are waiting for a spot in another group, but most of whom are not.

Another group that emerged was a group of severely symptomatic CSS clients who had substance abuse problems but who were unable to tolerate groups. One MICA staff member who was a social work student in group work started a six-week psychoeducation mini-group. There were three referrals to this "group," and two of the three showed up and continued to meet with this staff member once a week for 30 minutes in a very low stimulation setting. These two members were able to form a bond with each other and made progress in learning how substances impacted on their mental illness. It was originally hoped that these two clients would slowly be integrated into one of the larger MICA groups. In this case, these two members remained too fragile for a more intense group experience.

The program coordinator wanted a family psychoeducation service started for MICA families and significant others. The social work student expressed an interest in this. She had a strong background in multiple family psychoeducation groups and started a six-week series open to family members, significant others, and consumers of MICA services. This group ended with a self-help group organizer coming in to assist the family members with starting their own MICA family member self-help group.

One of the full-program members started a self help group for MICA consumers in October 1992. He succeeded in getting this meeting officially affiliated with NA. It meets three times a week, is well attended, and dually diagnosed clients openly discuss issues related to their mental illnesses as well as their substance abuse.

At this point, what one might call its toddlerhood, several dilemmas emerged. The program consisted of a first-step group and a full program, a multiple-family group, and minigroups for those MICA consumers unable to tolerate the stimulation of the larger groups. MICA clients who wanted MICA treatment were being served. However,

1. How could we be sure clients were getting the basic information and skills they needed to
   A. become or remain substance-free,
   B. lower hospital recidivism,
   C. experience fewer psychiatric exacerbations,
   D. live a higher quality of life?
2. When do you graduate from the MICA program? How can participants feel that they have completed a phase of treatment?
3. What are the criteria for moving on to the next step in recovery?
4. What do we do when a group member gets well enough to get employment, but still needs MICA treatment?

5. Are there some clients who stay in MICA treatment for the duration of their lives? If so, will this be the program that will provide that service?

The MICA staff began looking at all of these questions. By rearranging the groups, a more fully developed middle stage of programming has been implemented. This is a one-year modular series of group lectures and experientials that have a progressive educational focus as well as an emphasis on group interaction and skill building. Members will complete this series and will either end their MICA program involvement, or go into either the drop-in group if they want continued education and less of a commitment, or the new "recovery group" if they meet the membership criteria. The module will give the participant a sense of completion. It will assure the staff that needed information and skill building as well as a group support system have been offered in an organized and inclusive manner. (Information about the module can be obtained by writing to the author.)

Another change that has taken place is in the full program. The members have slowly become more able to use group process as a form of treatment and support network formation. They have been asking for more confrontation from each other and want to follow a theme through from one group to the next. As members became healthier and more self-assured, they came to claim the groups more for themselves. What started out as the full program evolved into a recovery group. The facilitators remain very active in their roles, but the groups are becoming more and more self-determined. The staff views this as a very positive outcome of MICA treatment at this level. Recovery members have come up with their own purpose of the group and criteria for membership.

Purpose:

1. to work toward recovery
2. to help each other survive and grow
3. to support each other through addiction and illness
4. to work on issues
5. to form bonds and create a nurturing social network
6. to develop trust

7. to offer feedback on issues of mental illness and drugs and alcohol
8. to learn to apply concepts to life as well as the group
9. to learn coping strategies

Criteria for membership:

1. to want recovery
2. to be working toward being symptom-free from mental illness
3. to be working toward being alcohol- and drug-free, with the exception of all prescribed drugs
4. to have a desire to participate in the purpose of the group
5. to have a willingness to engage in emotionally mature behavior during meetings
6. to have a commitment to group (being there)
7. to have a commitment to self-improvement
8. to have the ability to bond with group members
9. to have a willingness to share with group members
10. to be willing and able to accept group feedback
11. to have an ability to be honest

There has been discussion among staff regarding the need for a once or twice monthly aftercare group. There are several MICA group members who have day jobs or school hours that conflict with MICA groups. For the most part, these consumers have reached a level of stability that enables them to contribute to their communities in this way, but, it is felt that they are still in need of MICA group support.

THE PROGRAM AS IT STANDS NOW
(PREADOLESCENCE)

Four Phases of MICA Treatment

The ideal use of this system is to match the MICA consumer with the level of treatment that will best meet his or her needs. The consumer may move through the next phases of treatment as skill levels develop.

Phase I MICA Group Treatment

Criteria: The consumer

1. admits to the use of substances
2. is unable to tolerate group mode due to psychiatric symptoms

Purpose:

1. To educate the consumer about issues related to substance use and mental illness
2. To introduce the consumer to MICA treatment
3. To offer an opportunity to meet with one or two other MICA consumers in a time-limited small group experience

Structure/Method:

- One facilitator meets with small group once per week for 45 minutes for a prescribed period of weeks in a low-stimulation environment.
- Group is closed.
- The approach is didactic and concrete.
- Sharing of experiences/trust building is encouraged.

Phase II MICA Group Treatment (Drop-in)

Criteria: The consumer

1. is willing to explore the possibility that substance abuse may interfere with personal life goals
2. does not need to make a commitment to abstinence
3. is able to tolerate being a member of a group

Purpose:

1. To educate MICA consumers about mental illness and substance abuse
2. To provide a support network

Structure/Method:

- Cofacilitators meet with the group once per week for one hour.
- Group is ongoing absorbing new members as they are referred.
- Approach is didactic and educational.
- Minimum commitment to one group a month is needed.
- Group interaction is encouraged but not mandatory.
- Members are encouraged to attend community self-help groups.
- "Random" urine drug screenings once monthly.
- Breathalizing just prior to each meeting.

Phase III MICA Group Treatment (MICA Study)

Criteria: The consumer

1. is attempting to achieve abstinence
2. is able to tolerate a group
3. makes a commitment to attend each group

Purpose:

1. To provide a body of information related to mental illness and substance abuse and their interactions
2. To help each participant to understand how this body of knowledge relates to him or her personally and to other group members
3. To provide a process group for the discussion of member concerns
4. To explore coping skills for early recovery
5. To provide the beginnings of a sober support network

Structure/Method:

- Cofacilitators meet with the group two days per week; for one hour one day and for two hours the second day.
- Groups include one didactic, educational group and one experiential group (both based on modules created by MICA team members), and one process/support group per week.

- Verbal participation is stressed in both types of groups.
- Attendance in community self-help groups is stressed.
- "Soft" confrontation is encouraged.
- "Random" urine drug screening once per month.
- Breathalizing just prior to each meeting.

Phase IV MICA Group Treatment (Recovery)

Criteria: The consumer:

1. has been clean and sober at least six months
2. has a serious commitment to abstinence
3. has a knowledge of psychiatric symptoms
4. commits to attend each group
5. is engaged in an effective mental health program
6. agrees to participate fully in group
7. is able to take the risks involved in group intimacy

Purpose:

1. To provide a safe environment for the dually diagnosed consumer to explore the issues and skills of coping in a sober life-style
2. To encourage supportive, open relationships with others who have similar concerns and issues

Structure/Method:

- A one-hour meeting once a week with two coleaders.
- Occasional admission of a new member graduating from Phase III.
- Group process/mutual aid.
- Member-chosen topics.
- Attendance at community self-help is strongly encouraged.
- "Random" urine drug screening once each month.
- Breathalizing just prior to each meeting.

Phases of MICA Treatment–Addendum

Also offered are dual disorder staff-assisted self-help groups (the STEMSS model).

One of the "recovery" clients started a MICA self-help group (Twice Blessed) in the community. It is NA affiliated as a special-interest group.

A multiple-family group is offered twice a year for a series of eight meetings. All family members, significant others, and friends, as well as MICA consumers, are invited to this psychoeducation/support group.

The latest development is the addition of a fourth hour of group for those attending the Phase III MICA study group. This group will focus on "special topics." These topics will be chosen by both clients and staff.

It is interesting to look at the expectations that staff and agency had for MICA clients as the concept of MICA was first being acknowledged. There was little expectation that these service consumers would be able to tolerate or benefit from treatment. The reality is that a look at the evolution of the MICA program in its various stages and identifications of needs demonstrates not only the MICA client's ability to respond to treatment but an ability to state what the needs in treatment are. Members have been able to commit themselves to an appropriate level of treatment and to their fellow group members. Many of these consumers have not had a support network since their illnesses struck. Many of them are capable of attaining the MICA treatment goals of fewer hospitalizations, reduced relapse rates of both illnesses, increased social interaction and higher quality of life, and increased independent functioning in the community. This can be accomplished by offering a specifically tailored, multiphase MICA group program as part of a comprehensive outpatient treatment plan.

WHAT WORKS

What seems to work is relevant psychoeducation, structure, the development of and acceptance by a peer group, and the message that participants are capable of managing their illnesses. The elements of time and flexibility seem significant as well. It takes a long time under the best of circumstances for this population to learn to develop trust in one another. Relapse of either illness is not the end of treatment or even a failure. There are valuable lessons to be learned about one's self and other group members when relapse has occurred. The skills of both mental health workers and substance abuse workers need to be thoroughly discussed and integrated into an approach that is appropriate for each phase of treatment. It appears that the beginning treatment levels do better utilizing the mental health skills (for the severely mentally ill) of trust building, low stimulation, nonconfrontation, and psychoeducation. As treatment progresses, and egos become stronger, the introduction of more traditional substance abuse techniques, such as confrontation and group process, are effective in taking the client to the next level of competence in treatment. It will be interesting to watch and participate in the continuing development of MICA services. The path from conception to preadolescence has been stimulating, challenging, and rewarding. As MICA consumers continue to show us the way, the program will gradually develop into its adulthood.

REFERENCES

Aliesan, K. and Firth, R. C. (1990). A MICA program: Outpatient rehabilitation services for individuals with concurrent mental illness and chemical abuse disorders. *Journal of Applied Rehabilitation Counseling, 21*, 25-28.

Attia, P. R., (1988). Dual diagnosis: Definition and treatment. *Alcoholism Treatment Quarterly, 5*(3/4), 53-63.

Bauer, A. (1987). Dual diagnosis patients: The state of the problem. *Tie Lines.* IV(3), 1-4.

Carey, K. B. (1989). Treatment of the mentally ill chemical abuser: Description of the Hutchings day treatment program. *Psychiatric Quarterly,* Winter, 1-12.

Carey, M. P., Carey, K. B., and Meisler, M. S. (1991). Psychiatric symptoms in mentally ill chemical abusers. *The Journal of Nervous and Mental Disease, 170*(5), 136-138.

Drake, R. E., Antosca, L. M., Noordsy, D. L., Portals, S. D., and Osher, F. C. (1991). New Hampshire's specialized services for the dually diagnosed. In *New Directions for Mental Health Services*. Minkoff and Drake (Eds.) 50, 57-69.

Drake, R. E. and Wallach, M. A. (1989). Substance abuse among the chronic mentally ill. *Hospital and Community Psychiatry, 40* (10), 1041-1045.

Drake, R.E., McLaughlin, P., Pepper, B., and Minkoff, K. (1991). Dual diagnosis of major mental illness and substance disorder: An overview. In *New Directions for Mental Health Services*. 50, 3-12.

Flowers, J. V. and Booraem, C. T. (1991). A psychoeducational group for clients with heterogeneous problems: Process and outcome. *Small Group Research, 22*(2), 258-273.

Hanson, M., Kramer, T. H., and Gross, W. (1990). Outpatient treatment of adults with coexisting substance use and mental disorders. *Journal of Substance Abuse Treatment, 7,* 109-116.

Kaufman, E. (1989). The psychotherapy of dually diagnosed patients. *Journal of Substance Abuse Treatment, 6,* 9-17.

Lehman, A. F., Myers, C. P., and Corty, E. (1989). Assessment and classification of patients with psychiatric and substance abuse syndromes. *Hospital and Community Psychiatry, 40*(10), 1019-1024.

McKelvy, M. J., Kane, J. S., and Kellison, K. (1987). Substance abuse and mental illness: Double trouble. *Journal of Psychosocial Nursing, 25*(1), 20-25.

Minkoff, K. (1989). An integrated treatment model for dual diagnosis of psychosis and addiction. *Hospital and Community Psychiatry, 40*(10), 1031-1036.

Osher, F. C. and Kofoed, L. L. (1989). Treatment of patients with psychiatric and psychoactive substance abuse disorders. *Hospital and Community Psychiatry, 40*(10), 1025-1030.

Pepper B. and Ryglewicz, H. (eds). (1984). Advances in treating the young adult chronic patient. *New Directions For Mental Health Services, 21,* 91-113.

Reilly, P. G. (1987). Assessment and treatment of the mentally ill chemical abuser and the family. *Journal of Chemical Dependency Treatment, 4,* (1). 167-178.

Ridgely, M. S., Goldman, H. H., and Willenbring, M. (1990). Barriers to the care of persons with dual diagnoses: Organizational and financing issues. *Schizophrenia Bulletin, 16,* (1).

Ries, R. K. and Ellingson, T. (1990). A pilot assessment at one month of 17 dual diagnosis patients. *Hospital and Community Psychiatry, 41* (11), 1230-1233.

Ryglewicz, H. (1989). *Alcohol and Street Drugs: Time For A Choice* NY, TIE Inc.

Sciacca, K. (1987). New initiatives in the treatment of the chronic patient with alcohol/substance use problems. Tie Lines. IV (3), 5-6.

_____. (1991). An integrated treatment approach for severely mentally ill individuals with substance disorders. In *New Directions for Mental Health Services.* Minkoff and Drake (Eds.) 50, 69-84.

Test, M. A. (1981). Effective community treatment of the chronically mentally ill: What is necessary? *Journal of Social Issues, 37*(3), 71-83.

Thacker, W. and Tremaine, L. (1989). Systems issues in serving the mentally ill chemical abuser: Virginia's experience. *Hospital and Community Psychiatry, 40*(10), 1046-1049.

Zweben, J. E. and Smith, D. E. (1989). Considerations in using psychotropic medications with dual diagnosis patients in recovery. *Journal of Psychoactive Drugs, 21*(2), 221-228.

Chapter 18

From AA to A/CDFA: An Innovative 12-Step Model for Adult Children from Dysfunctional Family Backgrounds

Harle Thomas

INTRODUCTION

There can be no doubt that the Alcoholics Anonymous (AA) mutual aid group movement is one of the most significant social phenomena of the twentieth century (Bradshaw, 1988). With group meetings in every city in North America and an equally astounding number of meetings throughout the world, AA has earned the attention and respect of everyone involved in health services. For many, AA has come to represent the prototype of what a mutual aid group should be; its format and organization typify simplicity, economy, and centrality of purpose. AA has spawned a host of similarly formatted groups that identify with compulsive/addictive behaviors other than alcoholism; for example, NA, CA, GA, OA, and SA, which are groups for those struggling with the overuse or abuse of narcotics, cocaine, gambling, eating, and sex.

AA has grown in depth as well as in breadth through the establishment of groups for those who have been the nonabusive survivor of alcoholism: Al-Anon, for the nonabusive spouse or partner; Alateen, for the adolescents living in an alcoholic family situation; and ACOA, for adult children of alcoholics (that is, those adults who survived a childhood where alcoholism was present). These groups in turn have created models for similar support groups such as Nar-Anon, Co-Anon, Gam-Anon, and so forth.

While the impressive capacity to attract new members and the "cloning" facility of the AA model can be considered two of the group's great strengths, it can also be said that these attributes have legitimized the AA organizational plan and 12-step credo to the extent that many members of society now believe that there is only one way to "get recovery right" and only one sure way a mutual aid recovery group can be considered authentic and trustworthy–the "AA" way. To suggest another plan is to risk being seen as deviating from the norm by the "true" membership of AA groups (Davis Kasl, 1990).

And so the evolution of A/CDFA (a 12-step mutual aid group, Adult/Children of Dysfunctional Families Anonymous) not only describes the formation of a new self-help recovery group, but also exemplifies the process of one group's weaning away from those aspects of the AA groups model that were perceived by members of A/CDFA as rigid and patriarchal. These aspects will be examined further in this chapter; but to begin, a demonstration of the similarities between the groups will help to show some of the basic foundations that these two groups and many other mutual aid groups have in common.

SIMILARITIES OF THE AA MODEL
AND THE A/CDFA MODEL

1. Nonprofessional Support

The sense of *trust* through mutuality is one of the primary attractions of self-help/mutual aid groups. There is no power differential and no "ultimate authority" among the members, and for newcomers who are entering these groups in a great deal of conflict or confusion, this sense of equal footing can be most reassuring. This is not to suggest that self-help/mutual aid recovery groups are exclusionary alternatives to professional therapy. One assumption is that many members come to accept both professional and nonprofessional support during some stages of their recovery work with the understanding that issues can arise in recovery that are better treated under professional supervision.

However, some people simply cannot afford professional help. The vicissitudes of present-day economics and the cost of professional individual or group therapy make mutual aid groups (which are almost always free of cost) acceptable and desirable alternatives to no support at all. Further, some group members are justifiably apprehensive of one-on-one therapy and the risk inherent in unsupervised therapy situations. The growing interest in the support group "Stop ABC–Stop Abuse by Counselors," which has been established for clients who have been sexually abused by their professional therapists, exemplifies this apprehension.

2. Common Identity

The common element typically is the center of focus within the group; for example, alcoholics center on issues of alcoholism. The essence of mutuality is usually defined by some statement of purpose, such as the 12 Steps in AA or in A/CDFA. Other groups may have a mission statement, a set of guidelines, or a selection of readings that all members can identify with at a meaningful level.

The 12 Steps, however, are more than a statement that identifies its members. The 12 Steps also identify a process of self-exploration and spiritual discovery that form the basic process of recovery as defined by these groups. Put simply, the member may progress through the steps (at that member's own pace) from the initial acceptance of spiritual energy, through steps of self-exploration, to actual deeds of service that perpetuate recovery and engender new levels of discovery within the individual.

3. Shared Experience

This concept is the theoretical underpinning of the term "mutual aid." In AA and A/CDFA this sharing process is the sine qua non of the groups' existence. And because a meeting would not be a meeting without a substantial focus on sharing, several norms have been established.

Foremost among these norms is the one called "no crosstalk." Crosstalking occurs when a member of the group interrupts another member's sharing or speaks about that person's sharing when that person has finished. AA and A/CDFA recovery groups endorse the guideline that no one may interrupt, advise, confront, or question another person's sharing. This ensures safety from a variety of issues for both the sharer (who might feel diminished or threatened) and the crosstalker (who may be working through codependency or other interpersonal control issues). Only the sharer may talk; the others witness in empathetic silence. The no-crosstalk norm permits silences in the meetings on the assumption that there is a great power in attending silent witness as both an intervention and as an agent of change.

A second important guideline is that the person speaks in the "I/me" form. The focus is on expressing one's own feelings, attitudes, and responses to life experiences, rather than on commenting on the attitudes and behaviors of others. This can be seen both as a means to continue the process of self-exploration (self-help), and as a way to share one's own experience with the group (mutual aid).

Recovery groups believe that talking about one's own experience is an important step toward self-discovery; experience has a holistic sense to it. One is not just sharing anecdotes, but one is safe to experience feelings, memories, and sensations in the course of sharing in mutual aid groups. For many, feelings have been consistently or chronically repressed or depressed, and so experiential sharing can have a liberating and integrating sense to it (Miller, 1981, 1986).

Bowden and Gravitz (1985) put it succinctly, "If you feel safe, you will trust. If you trust, you will share. If you share, you will express your feelings. If you express your feelings, you will discover yourself. As you discover yourself, you *will* recover."

4. Anonymity

This concept is particularly described in the names of 12-step groups (they all end with anonymous). Not all mutual aid groups necessarily have to be anonymous, but in recovery groups, members' first names are typically the only means of personal identification. Again, safety is an important factor in this concept. Safety builds trust and trust builds capacity to share, feel, self-express, self-discover, and so on.

Anonymity may also be included in describing group membership, which is typically very fluid. Members come and go, some are "regulars," others drift in and out, making meetings larger one week, then smaller the next. What would seem exasperating in any task-oriented organization seems to work amazingly well in recovery-type support groups. The underlying statement is that there is no pressure to join or to keep coming back; this group is in no particular hurry to go anywhere or prove anything. There is, as in all groups, either a central contact person or a relatively consistent "core group," but the group formation itself is more or less "anonymous" inasmuch as the group may well be made up of different members from meeting to meeting. However, it is important to recognize that "anonymity" of members need not represent the surrendering of personal responsibility on some level for the development of the group.

These concepts help to give an overview of how 12-step recovery philosophy approaches self-help/mutual aid group organization. There are certainly more similarities, but these four are among the most basic and should give a fair impression of the nature of these groups.

Having said that, this chapter will now look at constructs that have caused an evolutionary process to occur within the self-help movement and in particular between AA, which has changed very little since its inception in the 1930s, and A/CDFA, which presents a more progressive model of a 12-step recovery group. The following differences will show an evolution or individuation process in which recent social attitudes have given rise to a reappraisal and reapplication of the basic AA tenets to allow for more validation of cultural and spiritual diversity.

DIFFERENCES BETWEEN THE AA MODEL
AND THE A/CDFA MODEL

1. Character-Disordered versus Neurotic-Based Approach

This is, perhaps, *the* central dividing line between AA, Al-Anon, ACOA, etc., on the one side, and A/CDFA on the other. Put simply,

A/CDFA supports the premise that methods that treat character-disordered people are inappropriate for the treatment of neurotically based people. A broader description of these terms will help clarify this discussion.

M. Scott Peck (1978) offered an interesting examination of character-disordered people and neurotically based people that can be applied to organizational approaches in recovery groups. In general, he posited, character-disordered people respond to their own self-created abusive crises by blaming others for the situation. A statement such as "If it weren't for this lousy job (etc.), I wouldn't have to drink so much" demonstrates the degree of unwillingness on the part of the character-disordered person to take responsibility for his/her own actions.

Contrasting with this description is the neurotically based person whose personal boundaries have been so chronically violated and broken down that, in response to having survived someone else's abusive behavior, the survivor will blame herself/himself. "If only I were a better wife (etc.), he wouldn't have this drinking problem" designates a person who is all too willing to blame herself/himself for someone else's abusive behavior.

A continuum is necessary to encompass the varying degrees of acceptance of responsibility; such a range allows for the complexity of human personality. Many people in recovery have aspects of both character-disordered and neurotically based responses to the way they experience life; there are members of support groups who are, at the same time, survivors and perpetrators of abusive behavior. But the degree to which a person is abusive should indicate the type of support group that would be most effective. It is not difficult to see that the more character-disordered person would benefit from a group whose format obliges the participant to see more clearly the impact of his/her abusive behavior and to take more responsibility for discontinuing it. On the other hand, for the more neurotically based personality, taking such responsibility would be contradictory to a sound recovery approach.

When looking at the array of recovery groups and the variety of members who are seeking mutual aid, this contrast between personality types has serious implications. For example, AA, NA, CA, SA, GA, etc., are frequented by character-disordered people. They fall into this general category because: (a) they are chronic abusers (they abuse the substance or experience in question, they abuse the others who live with them, they abuse themselves), and (b) they have difficulty taking responsibility for their actions. They may be remorseful, apologetic, and make conciliatory statements, but if they are chronically repeating the abuse, they have not yet taken real responsibility for ending the abuse and changing their behavior.

Going further with AA-type groups, an examination of the steps yields a description of the AA approach. Step 1 says, "We admitted we were *powerless . . . ;*" this helps to break through rigid egocentric defenses. Steps 2 and 3 have the member yield to the power of God; this also helps to break through the egocentric defenses. Step 4 has the member make a "fearless moral inventory" for all "character defects;" this encourages taking responsibility for one's actions. Step 5 continues by having the member admit the abuses (typically done privately with a seasoned member known as a sponsor); this also encourages taking responsibility for abusive behavior. Steps 8 and 9 have the member further take responsibility for his/her actions by making amends to people who were recipients of the abuse. Step 10 maintains this system by stating, "We continued to take a moral inventory of ourselves and when we were *wrong,* promptly admitted it." (Emphasis added.) This is an excellent and consistent approach to help chronic abusers break their addictive cycles.

However, these steps are not indicated for those who are survivors of the abuse. The fact that Al-Anon and ACOA and the entire range of Al-Anon "cloned" groups for survivors of abuse still use the AA steps with only minor alterations is thought of by A/CDFA as inappropriate and perhaps deleterious to the health of these members.

Consider, for example, what an SIA (Survivors of Incest Anonymous–an AA clone group) member must go through to admit in Step 1 that she/he is *"powerless."* This, after a childhood of powerlessness! Imagine having to believe in "God, as we understood *Him"* (as it was originally written before its recent upgrade to Him or Her). The majority of girls and boys who survived childhood sexual abuse were victimized by their fathers or stepfathers!

Ms. A., a 40-year-old member of A/CDFA, had been sexually abused as a child by her father and grandfather, and she had been dissuaded from exposing the situation by both her priest and her guidance counselor. Ms. A. associates words such as "God" or "Higher Power" with images of an omnipotent and controlling male figure. "Religion" conjures visions of imprisonment.

Why should a survivor make a "fearless moral inventory" as in Step 4 (for a neurotically based person, such a list might go on for pages), or make amends as in Steps 8 and 9, or promptly admit she or he was wrong, as in Step 10? There is no goodness of fit here.

Historically, A/CDFA diverged from ACOA in 1989 after the author of this chapter, along with a small group of ACOA members, came to the conclusion that while the spirit of the 12 Steps was a blessing to all in self-help recovery, in practice the process of the steps for a survivor-based population was unsuitable. In A/CDFA the steps eventually came to be adapted from the Charlotte Davis Kasl (1990) model and rewritten by the members themselves (as were the original AA 12 Steps written by Dr. Bob and Bill W. and their small group of recovering alcoholics). (See Figure 18.1.)

The A/CDFA 12 Steps reflect empowerment: Step 1 " . . . we have the power to change our lives and stop being dependent on others for our self-esteem and security." The emphasis here being to make use of what power one has, instead of taking away what little power one may have left. Steps 2 and 3 reflect empowerment both from within and without. Step 4 gives members the "context" of "multigenerational" cycles of behavior with which to examine their pasts. Step 6 helps a member "admit to her/his talents and accomplishments." Step 10 declares " . . . when we were *right*, we promptly admitted it." This innovative design for the 12 Steps has been interpreted by some members of AA groups as a controversial departure from the program.

2. God versus Recovery Resource(s)

The "God/Him" controversy has been aflame for many years in ACOA circles. There has been a reluctance to value other ways of understanding spirituality. It could be argued that the AA 12 Steps have been "legitimized" to the extent that they have become a cultural icon (Berger and Luckmann, 1966); the AA 12 Steps can be

FIGURE 18.1

THE TWELVE STEPS
for
ADULT/CHILDREN OF DYSFUNCTIONAL FAMILIES
Adapted from the 12-step model of Charlotte Davis Kasl (1990)
by the members of the A/CDFA Group, Montreal

1. We acknowledged we were in conflict because of our adult/child issues, but that we have the power to take charge of our lives and stop being dependent on others for our self-esteem and security.
2. Came to have faith that healing wisdom would be awakened within each of us if we opened ourselves to that power.
3. Declared ourselves willing to tune into our inner wisdom, to listen and act based upon faith in the truths of steps 1 and 2.
4. We examined our behaviors and beliefs in the context of living in a complex world of multigenerational family dysfunctions.
5. We shared with others the ways we have been harmed, harmed ourselves and others, striving to forgive ourselves and to change our behavior.
6. We admitted to our talents, strengths, and accomplishments, agreeing not to hide these qualities to protect others' egos.
7. Sought to strengthen our faith in the unconditional love of healing wisdom both within us and without us.
8. We became willing to let go of our shame, guilt, and any behavior that prevents us from taking control of our lives and loving ourselves.
9. We took steps to clear out all negative feelings between ourselves and other people by sharing grievances in a respectful way and making amends when appropriate.
10. Continued to trust our reality, and when we were right, promptly admitted it, affirming that we will no longer take responsibility for, analyze, or cover up the shortcomings of others.
11. Sought through prayer, meditation, and inner awareness to improve our ability to listen to our inward calling and gain the will and wisdom to carry that out.
12. Having had a spiritual awakening as the result of these steps, we tried to carry this message to other adult/children of dysfunctional families, and to practice these principles in all our affairs.

treated like scripture by many adherents of "fundamentalist AA-ism." This is unfortunate, especially when considering the internal conflict that may be engendered when recovering people who were sexually abused by their fathers or father figures have to believe in "God, as we understood Him" ("God/Him") in order to "get with the program."

More recently, Al-Anon and other AA derivative groups such as ACOA have evolved to using "God/God" (as opposed to "God/Him") and then "Higher Power/Higher Power," and this has been seen as a positive beginning. Sadly, these changes have been seen by many as a final concession. Again, Davis Kasl (1990) posits that this concept of God/Higher Power is a thinly guised androcentric patriarchal construct. That is, God has enjoyed anthropomorphic personification for so long that it feels awkward to consider God anything other than masculine. The words "higher" and "power" are two "masculine" interpretations of spirit as well. She goes on to say that many people, particularly women, view spiritual energy as "surrounding and transcending," being neither a higher nor even a single entity. This difference must be valued.

Peck (1978), in *The Road Less Traveled,* proposed that children tend to view "God" based on the conditions of their childhood relationships with their parents. He went on to suggest that children from dysfunctional family backgrounds invariably tend to see God as punishing, vengeful, or menacingly retributive. "God," as a word, is extremely value-laden, with so many sociolinguistic properties that it becomes problematic to use it safely within survivor-type recovery groups. "God" can be a "trigger" word, evoking feelings of powerlessness and worthlessness. The author of this paper has witnessed this reaction when discussions about the nature of "God" have been broached in ACOA and A/CDFA meetings that he has attended.

When ACOA literature spoke of "God" or "Higher Power," Mr. B. saw a white-robed, bearded giant of a man, omniscient and menacing, constantly threatening to hurl flaming thunder-bolts from above. Mr. B learned in his childhood that, try as hard as he might, he could never live up to impossible standards of the ideal son his father expected him to be. While

very successful in business, Mr. B.'s father was a heavy drink-
er and a hard taskmaster; he used beatings as a disciplinary
measure. Mr. B. always felt like a failure around him. Mr. B.
came to understand God as remote, judgmental, disapproving,
and disappointed; he continues to have a very deep resentment
toward "God, the Father." For many years Mr. B. "resolved"
the conflict by proclaiming himself an atheist.

Mr. B. said,

> Every time I felt I was getting into the ACOA group, a refer-
> ence to "God, the all-powerful, as I understood Him," became
> a great distraction. I had to expend a lot of energy to translate
> these words into something else so that I could hear the in-
> tended message. This limited my participation; I was strug-
> gling against my old definitions, images and feelings of worth-
> lessness which were constantly brought up in words like God
> and Higher Power.'

Often, a reference to God is one that can instill fear and resentment, as opposed to comfort, in those who have survived abuse
from parents in a dysfunctional family system. It is, therefore, an
important distinction when A/CDFA literature reads "recovery re-
source(s)" when discussing about spiritual energy. Recovery re-
source(s) is a neutral term that encompasses many different interpretations of spirituality. The (s) refers to Davis Kasl's point that,
while for many people all recovery resources are subsumed under
one single Resource, for others, there are many distinct resources.
The important point is that members in recovery groups share in
common a loss of faith, as Bradshaw (1988) calls it, "spiritual
bankruptcy," and it is therefore highly important to engender some
form of spiritual energy within each member without triggering
word images that reinforce negativism, powerlessness, and loss of
self-esteem.

3. Core Problems versus Manifestation

AA and AA-derivative groups focus on the specific addiction
and the management of its disuse: AA is for alcoholics, GA is for

gamblers, etc. There is a medical metaphor with a pathological bent to the AA approach. For example, the specific addiction is a disease; i.e., there is sickness and it can be treated through the draconian measure of total and complete abstinence. This reasoning, while tough to take for newcomers to the program, is highly effective in arresting chronic abuse.

However, there are at least two problems with this logic when it is applied to survivor groups. First, the metaphor that growing up in an abusive family has been like catching a contagious disease is endorsed in the literature. For example, in "The Problem" (an opening statement read at most ACOA meetings, ostensibly stating its purpose as helping ACOA's to identify with the common problem), there are lines such as the following:

> These symptoms of the family disease of alcoholism made us "co-victims"–those who take on the characteristics of the disease without necessarily ever taking a drink. . . . We either became alcoholics ourselves or married them or both. Failing that, we found another compulsive personality, such as a workaholic, to fulfill our *sick need* for abandonment. (ACOA, no publication date, emphasis added)

This type of literature reinforces a negative self-image. Again, while it may be considered by some to be an effective tool in abuser-type groups to break down rigid ego barriers, it is out of place when dealing with people whose egos have been shattered through suffering chronic abuse.

> Ms. C., after attending A/CDFA meetings for a while, shared a personal revelation at one meeting that she had always identified herself as sick, mentally ill, abnormal, and powerless. She expressed her gratitude for a group that, through its writing, emphasized and nurtured whole other aspects of her personality that she didn't believe she had. She said that by being in a group that endorsed the power of survivorship, the ability to grow from within, and the affirmation of talents and accomplishments, she was beginning to see herself in a new light. This new insight was manifested in Ms. C.'s increasing ability to make eye contact and interact more freely in the group.

Second, most survivors have an array of "symptoms." Many survivors come from families where addictions existed, some do not. Some were raised in families where the dysfunction was obvious, some were raised in families where the dysfunction was hidden behind rigid rules, control, and secrecy. Many survivors come from multiaddicted or polyabusive family backgrounds, presenting a complex assortment of interwoven survivor responses. This is to say that members of A/CDFA come from a wide assortment of family backgrounds, from life in multiple foster homes to growing up in a home where a parent died slowly of a long-term illness, to survivorship of childhoods where alcoholism, physical abuse, and/or incest was present. "Symptoms" are not the main common identifiers in A/CDFA groups.

A/CDFA does not focus on the management of disease symptoms; A/CDFA explores the core problems for the conflicts by which the survivors are challenged. A/CDFA supports Bradshaw's (1988) supposition that there are basically two core issues that face people in recovery: spiritual bankruptcy and low self-love. By examining ways of generating and enhancing faith and self-love, A/CDFA tends to focus on the underlying forces behind the compulsive, self-defeating behaviors.

The A/CDFA format incorporates practical ways of addressing these core problems. For example, A/CDFA provides time in its meetings to do affirmation work, to offer an exercise that may help members internalize positive messages about themselves that will compensate, if not replace, the many internalized negative messages from childhood. These meetings also include a brief time for meditation to generate a new sense of spiritual energy that is connected with the self.

Because a common identity is a crucial factor in a group's cohesion, any question of identity in a recovery group must address the extent to which the group identifies its members as "sick" or "well." Where A/CDFA and AA groups differ is that A/CDFA wants to replace negative self-image (survivors are diseased by contagion), with a more positive motivation to change (survivors have powers they are just now discovering they can use).

4. *Importance of Change and Choice Making*

It seems ironic that a recovery group such as AA is seemingly so reluctant to change within itself. One could argue that the AA model presents strong overtones of religious institutionalism: sponsors as confessors, the 12 Steps as a process of confession and atonement for sins, the AA literature as unalterable scripture, and AA's Central Service Board as a hierarchical council that sanctions which recovery books and literature are acceptable for members to read. As with other huge organizations, what appears as revolutionary in one period of time can appear ossified and conservative in a later period if it cannot keep abreast of the changing needs of the people it serves.

A/CDFA embraces and exalts change and choice making. There are many examples: the literature is contained in a loose-leaf notebook; it has not been paginated. At the end of each month, the group members present at the end of that meeting decide what pages are to be added or deleted from the notebook. In this way ownership of the meaningfulness of the readings rests on the judgment of the members presently in the group. That this group allows for its members' writing to be integrated into the meeting format has helped to provide empowerment for all members of the group and produces writing and thinking that is beneficial to recovery.

> Recently, the current members of A/CDFA chose to set aside the Opening and Closing readings in the A/CDFA notebooks for a six-week period. This choice allowed members to take responsibility for selecting new readings and by so doing to feel empowered and refreshed. More than a few of the writings are created by the members themselves. Mr. D. and Ms. E. are gifted writers who are able to capture the feelings, attitudes, and triumphs of many of the members of this group; their writings have a special meaning to comembers as such writing seems to focus appropriately on the current needs and attitudes of the group.

The point has been made previously that many mutual aid recovery groups are amorphous in membership definition, and so the literature tries to reflect the current needs of the group by putting faith in the choice making of its most current members. Many members bring in writings and poetry from other authors that they believe has particular meaning for the group.

Also, the group meeting has choice making built into it. Members select readings from the format, or they may bring in their own, or may give spontaneous testimony. What is significant here is that the members create the meeting. In AA there is a fairly rigid structure and a hierarchy of command, the top echelon of which sends sanctioned reading material to each of the groups. A/CDFA, with its independent status, tends to have considerably more immediacy among its members. This immediacy encourages change as well. A/CDFA believes that compulsion and choice making are mutually incompatible. People can get rid of the one by practicing the other.

CONCLUSION

In examining the formation and development of recovery-type self-help mutual aid groups, this paper has looked at the similarities and differences between the AA groups model and the A/CDFA model.

Their philosophical and practical approaches to recovery are similar in the importance placed on nonprofessional intervention, common identity, shared experience, and anonymity. The groups' philosophies differ in the metaphorical understanding of the nature of survivorship. The AA-groups model still tends to use the "disease," rigid ego-barrier breaking, character-disordered approach in its groups, while A/CDFA has progressed to identifying common core issues of spiritual bankruptcy and low self-love and creating self-help interventions that address those issues. A/CDFA also makes it a point to exalt and model the empowerment acquired by making choices and changes by virtue of the very organization of the group's literature and meeting format.

Throughout, there is one concept on which both groups strongly agree. Both groups recognize faith as the single most important milestone in recovery. Faith in the goodness of oneself, faith in the goodness of the group, and faith in the goodness of one's spirituality.

REFERENCES

ACOA (Current literature, no specified date). Literature package of ACOA. Torrance, CA: Central Service Board and Interim World Service Organization.

Berger, P. & Luckmann, T. (1966). *The social construction of reality.* Garden City, NY: Anchor Books.

Bowden, J. D. & Gravitz, H. L. (1985). *Recovery: A guide for adult children of alcoholics.* New York: Simon & Schuster.

Bradshaw, J. (1988). *Bradshaw on: Healing the shame that binds you.* Deerfield Beach, FL: Health Communications, Inc.

Davis Kasl, C. (1990). The twelve-step controversy. *Ms.* November/December, 30-31.

Miller, A. (1981). *The drama of the gifted child: The search for the true self.* New York: Basic Books.

_____. (1986). *Thou shalt not be aware: Society's betrayal of the child.* New York: Meridian Publishers.

Peck, M. S. (1978). *The road less traveled.* New York: Simon & Schuster.

Index

Differentiation group development
     stage, 118,149-150,162-163
Discrimination, 139-140
Disempowerment of women, 123,
     131,147,154
"Double Jeopardy," of minority
     culture elderly, 102
Dual-purpose group
  functional vs. instructional
     purpose of, 53-54,55
  implications, recommendations
     for
     dual-role relationships, 60-61
     education vs. therapy, 59-60
     field practicum, 59
     involuntary participation, 60
     peer leader's competence, 60
  misuse of
     dual-role relationships, 58-59
     education vs. therapy, 57
     field practicum substitution,
       56-57
     involuntary participation, 57-58
     peer-leader's competence, 58
  use of, 54-56
     learning cycle stages and, 54-55

Ecological social work, 68
Education, educators
  inferiority of, 67
  issues facing, 2
  vs. therapy, 57,59-60
  See also Cultural sensitivity skills
Elderly issues. *See* Vietnamese older
     people
Empathy
  in 12-step mutual aid groups, 246
  African-American issues and, 129
  in sexual offenders group
     treatment, 184-185,187
  in women's group development,
     120-121,123,127-129,136

Empirical Foundations of Group
     Work Practice Symposium,
     37
Empowerment
  of A/CDFA, 250,251,256
  of adult incest survivors, 191
  in debriefing nursing groups,
     162-163
  disempowerment of women
     and, 123,131,147,154
  of ethnic groups, 73,74,109,114
  feminist approach to, 147
  opportunities for, 38,43
  vs. oppression, 153
  of students, 77-79
  value of, 35
  See also Women in poverty
Environmental intervention, 35,36,
     43
ESAT Program. *See* Sexual offenders
     group treatment
Ethnic identity
  importance of, 73,74
  interethnic conflict and, 74,78
  See also Chinese society issues;
     Vietnamese older people;
     Women in poverty
Ethnocentrism dangers, 73
Etobicoke Adolescent Offenders
     Group. *See* Sexual offenders
     group treatment
Etobicoke Sexual Abuse Treatment
     (ESAT) Program. *See* Sexual
     offenders group treatment
European Group Work Symposium,
     37
Expressive ties relationships, 94,98n2

Face-saving (Chinese), 93,95,96-97
Facilitator. *See* Worker
Familial patriarchy, 140-141
Family. *See* Adult incest survivors;
     Adult/Children of
     Dysfunctional Families
     Anonymous (A/CDFA);